PRAISE FOR
Gifts in Dark Packages

"Catherine's book is a resilience instruction manual, but it reads like a conversation with a friend. Witty and wise, emotional and impactful, Catherine's storytelling takes you on a journey of self-exploration that will help you appreciate the peaks and valleys we all face and see them for the gifts they truly are. Add this book to your resilience toolbox immediately!"

— **Ian Tyson, Veteran Motivational Speaker, Author, Coach and Silver Lining Prospector**

Gifts in Dark Packages is, in a word, a gift. For anyone who has gone through dark days (and nights), the messages in the book are confirming, relevant and incredibly helpful. So many "how-to" books have a glib approach, offering us quick pronouncements about how to live a better life. Catherine's down-to-earth approach is different — it's real. Catherine's work as a trauma counsellor and corporate wellness coach has added perspective and insight to her well-laid-out formula for remaining mentally fit through the challenges life brings us (especially loss, change and disconnection). It reflects her lived experience and learnings. She writes about how easily we can go down a troubled path after experiencing significant stress. And how we can unwrap the gift of that trauma and rise through it to transform our lives.

— **M. Cole Cohen, Ph.D., Mental Health Leadership Pioneer and Key Architect of the Bell 'Let's Talk' and Queen's University Certificate Training Program for Leaders**

"A must-read! Catherine's roadmap to mental health resiliency is fresh, bold and greatly needed. The reader will be left with much-needed valuable tools to use when tackling all of life's great challenges."

— **Mike Shoreman, Motivational Speaker, Author, Wellness and Leadership Expert, Mental Health and Disability Advocate, and SUP Man of the Year 2020/2021**

"Catherine has a beautiful capacity to address complex topics with care, warmth and lightheartedness. This must-read book is rich with tangible tools for transformation and support as you reclaim your gifts and come home to yourself."

— **Marlee Liss, Sensuality Coach, Speaker and Restorative Justice Advocate**

"This important book comes at a critical time when we are all seeking the gift within adversity. Catherine makes the journey easy with her profound wisdom and vulnerable storytelling — captivating and comforting all at the same time. This book is the greatest gift."

— **Rina Rovinelli, 2020 Top 25 Women of Influence™, Co-Founder of Speaker Slam and Speaker Coach**

"I highly recommend this book for those who are looking for inspiration and motivation throughout their own life journey. Catherine has a gift for bringing life lessons alive in a refreshing manner that engages and influences both employees and leaders in the corporate setting — which easily sets her apart from others."

— **Rachel Turner, Senior Director Global Strategic Initiative and Integrations, TELUS International.**

GIFTS
IN DARK PACKAGES

How to Embrace Adversity,
Transform Your Life
and Experience Joy

Catherine Clark, M.Ed.

First published by Ultimate World Publishing 2022
Copyright © 2022 Catherine Clark

ISBN
Paperback: 978-1-922828-22-4
Ebook: 978-1-922828-23-1

Catherine Clark has asserted her rights under the Copyright, Designs and Patents Act 1988 to be identified as the author of this work. The information in this book is based on the author's experiences and opinions. The publisher specifically disclaims responsibility for any adverse consequences which may result from use of the information contained herein. Permission to use information has been sought by the author. Any breaches will be rectified in further editions of the book.

All rights reserved. No part of this publication may be reproduced, stored in or introduced into a retrieval system, or transmitted in any form, or by any means (electronic, mechanical, photocopying, recording or otherwise) without the prior written permission of the author. Any person who does any unauthorized act in relation to this publication may be liable to criminal prosecution and civil claims for damages. Enquiries should be made through the publisher.

Cover design: Nathalie Shnider
Layout and typesetting: Ultimate World Publishing

Ultimate World Publishing
Diamond Creek,
Victoria Australia 3089
www.writeabook.com.au

First and foremost, for all the brave souls who have yet to unwrap their dark gifts, I'm honoured to guide you on this transformational journey.

For my mother, Dorothy, the beautiful rose in whose soil I have my roots.

To my son, Andrew, my endless source of inspiration, and my daughter, Nathalie, my eternal ray of sunshine.

*"The dark night of the soul comes just before the revelation.
When everything is lost, and all seems darkness, then comes
the new life and all that is needed."*
— Joseph Campbell

CONTENTS

INTRODUCTION 1
THE ROADMAP 7

PART ONE

ACKNOWLEDGE YOUR GIFTS IN DARK PACKAGES ... 17
   CHECKPOINT 1: 19
      Hotel Saskatchewan Breakdown 20
      Feeling is Healing 23
      Making Mental Health Matter 35
      Rediscovering Your Resilient Hero 41
      Pondering Post-Traumatic Growth 46

PART TWO

ACCEPT YOUR GIFTS IN DARK PACKAGES 51
   CHECKPOINT 2: 53
      Aligning With Self-Acceptance 59
      Creating Space for Self-Compassion 65
      Finding Freedom in Self-Forgiveness 73
      Forgiving Others 78

PART THREE

EMBRACE YOUR GIFTS IN DARK PACKAGES 83
   CHECKPOINT 3: The Phoenix Fix 85
      Power of Self-Reflection 86

CHECKPOINT 4: Curb Your Catastrophizing 99
- Locus of Control 103
- Crooked Maladaptive Thinking 108
- Broaden and Build 113
- Toxic Positivity 114

CHECKPOINT 5: Surrender It All 117
- Mindfulness Meditation 120
- Morning Routine (RINGS) 134

CHECKPOINT 6: Off-Balance 141
- Loving Use of Time 142
- Work-Life Integration 145
- Boundaries 101 150
- Self-Care is Critical 153
- Self-Care Plan/Checklist 157

CHECKPOINT 7: Challenging Change 161
- Career Change 163
- Bridging Change 170
- Traumatic Change 174
- Grit and Growth Mindset 178

CHECKPOINT 8: Living Through Loss 185
- Gifts of Grief Unwrapped 189
- Getting Good at Grief 191
- Complicated Grief (Suicide, Miscarriage and Pet Loss) 198

CHECKPOINT 9: Deconstructing Disconnections — Cultivating Connections 201
- Human Connection Deficit Syndrome 203
- Relationship Disconnections — Out of the Dark 207
- Moving Forward — Unwrapping the Dark Gift 209
- Getting to Self-Love 212
- Self-Love is the New Sexy 220
- Cultivating Loving Friendships 222

CHECKPOINT 10: Daring Difficult Conversations 233
    Show Up Fully — Empathic Communication 241
    Expressing Yourself 246
    Be a Humorous Storyteller 248

PART FOUR

GIVE YOUR GIFTS IN DARK PACKAGES 253

    CHECKPOINT 11: Passion Meets Purpose —
    Living Your Dark Gifts 255

AFTERWORD – FINAL THOUGHTS 269
ACKNOWLEDGEMENTS 273
NOTES 277
REFLECTIONS 283
ABOUT THE AUTHOR 287

Disclaimer

I have written this book from my own personal and professional experience. Names and details have been altered where necessary to protect identities. When reading this book, if you feel triggered or if frightening feelings arise, please seek the help of a counsellor, medical professional or supportive trusted friend.

INTRODUCTION

"One does not become enlightened by imagining figures of light, but by making the darkness conscious."
— Carl Jung

Congratulations! By picking up this book, you've taken the first step towards living a life with greater ease and joy. You're stronger and more resilient than you think. You've chosen to go to a bookstore or seek help online instead of suffering in silence. You've decided to fully show up for YOU — for your beautiful soul. You're finally ready to stop struggling.

Admit it: the jig is up.

You don't have the strength to keep on playing the game and pretending like you have it all together. At the very least, you're probably suffering from imposter syndrome — doubting your skills and talents, thinking it was just luck that got you here. You feel undeserving of your success and have a persistent internalized fear of being exposed as a "fraud" and, soon enough, people will discover the truth about you.

That's where I was in the summer of 2019 when I found myself at my rock bottom: terrified, broken, bruised and barely functioning. I was drowning in a sea of self-deception, praying for a life preserver to be tossed my way. By day, I masqueraded as a competent mental health professional with a full schedule of corporate wellness workshops. By night, I was a mental health disaster — my personal life had completely unravelled. I was petrified of being exposed for all my incompetence and failure. Perfectionism and superhuman controlling of, well, everything, hadn't kept me safe from harm.

This time, my dark package was the end of my second marriage, which imploded catastrophically — I'd been living a lie for twenty-three years. My inner circle of trusted advisors, including my psychotherapist, knew a full-blown breakdown was imminent. On November 1, 2019, I bought a ticket to the beautiful Sunshine Coast of British Columbia, Canada and checked myself into a spiritual retreat center. I knew I could no longer keep up the charade. I was a zombie. I needed to be by the ocean — my grounding element. I needed to step into my pain, climb into the darkness, ask for help and finally use the mental health strategies I'd so freely offered to others.

The heartache, pain and anguish were only starting to dissipate when in March 2020, an upside-down Covid-19 tsunami hit, spreading apocalyptic fear and dread in its wake and leaving most of us sucker-punched and gasping for air.

Say what? The dark packages keep on coming! On top of everything else that happened this year, we can't socialize or even hug anymore? We could literally die, I thought, defeated.

By the fall of 2020, I had a resounding epiphany: *I am rising from this hellish quagmire. I am going to write a book. I have phenomenal coping strategies and resiliency tools — I just need to use them on myself and then show others how to do the same.*

So, here's my big secret: *I messed up really, really badly in my life.* I took the wrong jobs, stayed married to the wrong people and supported everyone else — all while acting as my own worst enemy. In fact, I became so skilled at self-sabotage and beating myself up that I should have won an Olympic boxing medal.

Here's my big self-honesty share: *I'm just as scared as you are.* At times it feels like there's no way out of the darkness, but I'm here to tell you there's a flashlight and a way forward. I found mine and you will find yours too.

This book is for anyone who feels stuck in their struggle to survive, or anyone with a friend, mother, father, sibling, daughter or son who can't see a path forward through their current life calamity. No matter what you're experiencing — job loss, miscarriage, death of a loved one — I want you to know you're not alone in your pain. It might feel insurmountable to you right now. That's normal. But I know by the time you finish this book you will have a Mental Health Resiliency Roadmap and the tools you need to feel better — live better. If you're at that dark, low, critical moment right now, you've already made a decision to feel better by simply picking up this book.

What follows are the stories I have been blessed to share about my tumultuous life, the mental health challenges of my clients and the real-life struggles of my friends. Stories of brokenness, betrayal and the bittersweet. Stories of how the darkest moments can shine a transformative light on any life.

My darkest packages first started showing up on my doorstep in my twenties — their unwelcome delivery prompted by the premature death of my father and several close friends, a life-threatening tumour, an abusive "sex addict" first husband and debilitating depression. I joined the "face your own mortality, no fear" club, but never fully unwrapped my dark gifts. So, they kept showing up.

On the outside, I appeared healed and busied myself with taking care of others. Truth be told, I was simply regifting these dark packages to others by doling out therapeutic advice, distracting myself from my own pain and negating any opportunity for real spiritual growth.

Bottom line: *You can run but you can never hide from your inner darkness. The things you try to avoid will just keep coming back.*

My most recent deliveries — marital, psychological and professional breakdowns — gave me the gift of time to reset. So, after the Covid-19 pandemic hit, I fell into my typical "help others" avoidance strategy. Without missing a beat, I launched Coffee with Catherine on Instagram — an IGTV channel offering strategies for improving mental wellness. And then it hit me — debilitating anxiety, a clear reminder that you need to put your oxygen mask on first before helping others. Even though it felt like I had to save the world, what I really needed was to save myself.

So, I finally, fully committed to finding my inner light: therapy, healthy eating, meditation, gratitude, exercise and financial literacy. I started journalling again, which reignited my desire to write. *Et voilà!* The book you're holding in your hands, all thanks to those dark moments.

So, the real question is: Were all these choices and experiences really mistakes? Or were they gifts — nuggets of learning — that have made me the resilient woman I am today?

I'm suggesting we put a new spin on our adversities — right here, right now, in the wide-open spaces of these pages. Why not flip our perspective and look at difficult moments as opportunities for invaluable insight for our soul's evolution? A way to reveal what you still need to heal in order to suffer less and enjoy life more. Let's call them "dark gifts."

Let's create a whole new mindset — "get unleashed," as author Elizabeth Gilbert refers to it in her book, *Big Magic (2016)*. Let's mobilize, galvanize and reignite our stories. Let's unwrap our dark packages and ask the tough questions we often avoid when tragedy strikes. Questions such as "How did I get here?" and "What is the inner wisdom in this dark package?" The pressure to achieve the perfect white-picket-fence life will continue to stalk you, knock you flat on your back and keep haunting you until you accept the gifts the universe has been trying to give you all along.

Think of me as the friend who sits beside you when you're staring at the bottom of a post-breakup Häagen-Dazs ice cream carton. The friend who also happens to have a trauma counselling background and can empathically say, "I hear your struggle. It's messy, it feels insurmountable, it's valid and I'm here for you." I'm the friend who wrote a book to help people who are struggling with their mental health and in the process confronted her own darkest shadows. I'm telling you the truth so that you too will have the courage to tell yourself the truth.

Life doesn't always turn out as we expect. It can be complex, rewarding, harsh, joyful, mean, hilarious and utterly perplexing. We are all beautifully human, flawed and vulnerable. To heal, we sometimes just need to give ourselves permission to sit in the dark puddle of pain — to feel really shitty without all the guilt and judgement. Let's be honest — personal growth and transformation is a messy process.

Everyone has their own pathway to healing, whether that be through yoga, cognitive behavioural therapy (CBT), martial arts or meditation, or something else. Unfortunately, I don't have a magic wand to get you there. But what I do have is extensive experience in navigating my own way, along with years of helping clients move through a minefield of very distressing, sometimes darkly humorous, situations.

I hope you'll share the stories of this road trip and these resiliency tools with your friends and family members so that they may also courageously rise and never settle for less than they deserve!

THE ROADMAP

*One day you finally knew
what you had to do, and began,
though the voices around you
kept shouting their bad advice –
though the whole house began to tremble
and you felt the old tug at your ankles.
"Mend my life!" each voice cried.
But you didn't stop.
You knew what you had to do,
Though the wind pried
With its stiff fingers
At the very foundations,
Though their melancholy was terrible.
It was already late enough,
and a wild night,
and the road full of fallen
branches and stones.
But little by little,
as you left their voice behind,
the stars began to burn*

*through the sheets of clouds,
and there was a new voice,
which you slowly recognized as your own,
that kept you company as you strode
deeper and deeper into the world,
determined to do the only thing you
could do –
Determine to save the only life
That you could save.*
— Mary Oliver, *The Journey*

So, are you ready?

Ready to start this journey? Ready to discover your greatest gift, that no one else on this earth possesses? The amazing YOU. Ready to build up your resiliency muscle and embrace the hidden gems of adversity buried deep in your dark packages?

You'll definitely need a good roadmap, so I've got you covered.

Keep in mind, as Pulitzer Prize-winning poet, Mary Oliver, describes in *The Journey (2020)*, it's not going to be an uneventful trip. There will be some bumpy patches and emotional upheaval. Leaving behind an unhealthy way of being and starting anew is never easy but think of this road trip as your own personal Hero's Journey — the journey from suffering to enlightenment that spiritual leaders have described for centuries. The same series of experiences that Joseph Campbell outlined in his 1949 book, *The Hero with a Thousand Faces (2008)*, that every individual goes through — whether you're Mother Teresa, Luke Skywalker or amazing *you*. You get to choose your own route and which dragons to slay along the way.

I begrudgingly began my mental health resiliency journey at the age of thirty, suffering from ill health and depression, immobilized by fear. I needed major surgery to remove a lime-sized tumour on my first rib. It had moved my trachea over an inch and caused my arm to go completely dead at night. The risks of surgery were extremely devastating — severed vocal cords, paralysis on the left side of the body and optic nerve damage — and I was told the tumour would eventually kill me, albeit painfully slowly. As if that was any consolation. So, what choice did I have? I soldiered on, had the risky thoracic surgery and, for all intents and purposes, it was a resounding success.

After the lab confirmed my tumour was benign non-cancerous, one of the first phone calls I received was from my dear friend and work colleague, Kathy. While pregnant with twins, she was diagnosed with stomach cancer and told she had less than a year to live. This was an unbelievably heart-wrenching situation. I've never felt so guilty in my life, telling someone I did not have cancer, as I did with Kathy that day. I could feel her spirit beaming on the other end of the phone as she said, "I'm so happy you have good news, Cath. There's so much you're meant to do in this lifetime. You're such a bright light!"

So, there I was, on the wide-open roadway of life, paralyzed by the enormity of my good fortune, unable to reconcile why a mother of twins would have her life cut short while I was allowed to live. That day marked the beginning of my spiritual awakening — breaking free of negative patterns and emotional pain — a lifelong journey I'm still on today.

Three decades later, I've incorporated all of this learning into a Mental Health Resiliency Roadmap to help you find your inner directional wisdom — your own truth — and do a hard reset on your GPS. A way to say yes to your gifts in dark packages amidst all the construction zones and detours life throws at us. As Mary Oliver suggests, it's a roadmap of self-discovery — amongst the tangled mess of fallen branches. The payoff is that you'll uncover your own faint little voice getting louder and clearer after being squelched by years of self-sabotage and bullying.

So, wherever you are on this life journey right now, we can share the same roadmap — the one I've been field testing for decades and will continue to refine for the rest of my life.

Let's hit the dusty trail.

It's okay if you feel hesitant — readiness can't be rushed or forced. Please know just sitting in your car with curiosity, an open mind and the roadmap in your hands is a great start. You can just listen to some tunes and study the map while you flip through the first few pages in this book. Take all the time you need.

When you're ready, I'll be right here. I still have lots of life lessons to learn and practise alongside you. We can travel along the road to mental health resiliency together — learning valuable and actionable tools at each checkpoint. The car is started, the tank is full and the road trip playlist is ready to go, so remember to enjoy the ride. Rest assured the tools found in the following pages will help you remove roadblocks, let go of what's no longer serving you and cruise along the highway home to the most amazing version of YOU.

There are eleven major checkpoints (⦿) I've plugged into the GPS for our Mental Health Resiliency Roadmap. Each checkpoint will align with the specific lessons and "self-oriented" traits that you'll need (e.g., self-awareness, self-honesty) to successfully navigate your way toward an "optimally thriving," flourishing YOU.

Why eleven? In numerology, eleven is considered a high vibrational number that signifies vision and self-fulfillment. The prime number 11 is also called "the teacher," thought to teach you important lessons for your life. As in the Hero's Journey, the Mental Health Resiliency Roadmap also has eleven stops on the road to transformation.

Eleven also represents finding emotional, spiritual and cognitive balance, which I believe you'll achieve as you travel along this path. The mental health resiliency tools provided will not only increase your ability to bounce forward from trauma and difficult situations, but they are also intended to prevent a downward spiral in the first place. They'll keep your car on the road, safely in drive.

Here are the eleven checkpoints on this road trip that are divided into four separate parts outlined below.

PART ONE: ACKNOWLEDGE

Look at your dark package, understand your emotional state, consider your mental health challenges and acknowledge the resilient hero within while gathering support along the way.

♀ CHECKPOINT 1 — *Self-Awareness and Self-Honesty*

PART TWO: ACCEPT

Make peace with yourself and your past.

♀ CHECKPOINT 2 — *Self-Acceptance, Self-Compassion and Self-Forgiveness*

PART THREE: EMBRACE
Discover teachable moments, identify resiliency tools you already possess and add mindset-shifting strategies for authentic transformation.

- **CHECKPOINT 3** — *Self-Reflection and Self-Observation*
- **CHECKPOINT 4** — *Self-Talk and Self-Esteem*
- **CHECKPOINT 5** — *Self-Surrender and Self-Knowing*
- **CHECKPOINT 6** — *Self-Discipline and Self-Care*
- **CHECKPOINT 7** — *Self-Clarity and Self-Transitioning*
- **CHECKPOINT 8** — *Self-Heal and Self-Soothe*
- **CHECKPOINT 9** — *Self-Love and Self-Sharing*
- **CHECKPOINT 10** — *Self-Belief and Self-Expression*

PART FOUR: GIVE
Where passion meets purpose. Give your dark gifts, live your legacy, serve your highest purpose and harness your unlimited potential so that you can simply enjoy life.

- **CHECKPOINT 11** — *Self-Enjoyment and Self-Fulfillment*

I suggest you start your road trip with a deep-dive at Part One, Checkpoint 1 to get a better understanding of your current emotional state — honour and validate what you've gone through in your life. You can also learn more about the possible resources you can use to address specific mental health concerns. Afterwards, fill your tank with the high-octane self-acceptance, self-compassion and self-forgiveness all found in Part Two, Checkpoint 2.

Thereafter, you may move through the checkpoints in Part Three in order, or choose those most pertinent to your current life challenges, because your journey is unique. You may start at one checkpoint then find you need to go back or skip ahead. Check the menu of dark packages to find what works best for you. There's no right or wrong route and the road less travelled is always available to you. You choose which checkpoints you need right now. Then read, rest and digest in whatever order makes you feel roadworthy in your life.

You can print out the Mental Health Resiliency Roadmap at www.catherineclarkconnects.com and post it on your bulletin board. That way you can track your own progress. Use the map to focus your attention on the tools you'll need to practise at any given time to shift your mindset, rise above adversity and live an easier life.

At each checkpoint, you'll find several exercises such as ☕ Coffee with Catherine, including coaching questions to prompt discussion as if we were sitting across from each other at a coffee shop or at a pit stop on our journey. I don't know about you, but I need to refuel with a good coffee and good conversation on a long road trip.

Of course, you'll also need to stop off at the gift shop and pick up some souvenirs. The gift shop is where you'll find what I call 🎁 Gift Box Resiliency Tools at each checkpoint exit. These are actionable steps for you to practise to solidify the self-oriented traits and skills you need to be more resilient and mentally healthy. They're the same resiliency techniques I've been providing in my wellness workshops and counselling sessions for over twenty-five years.

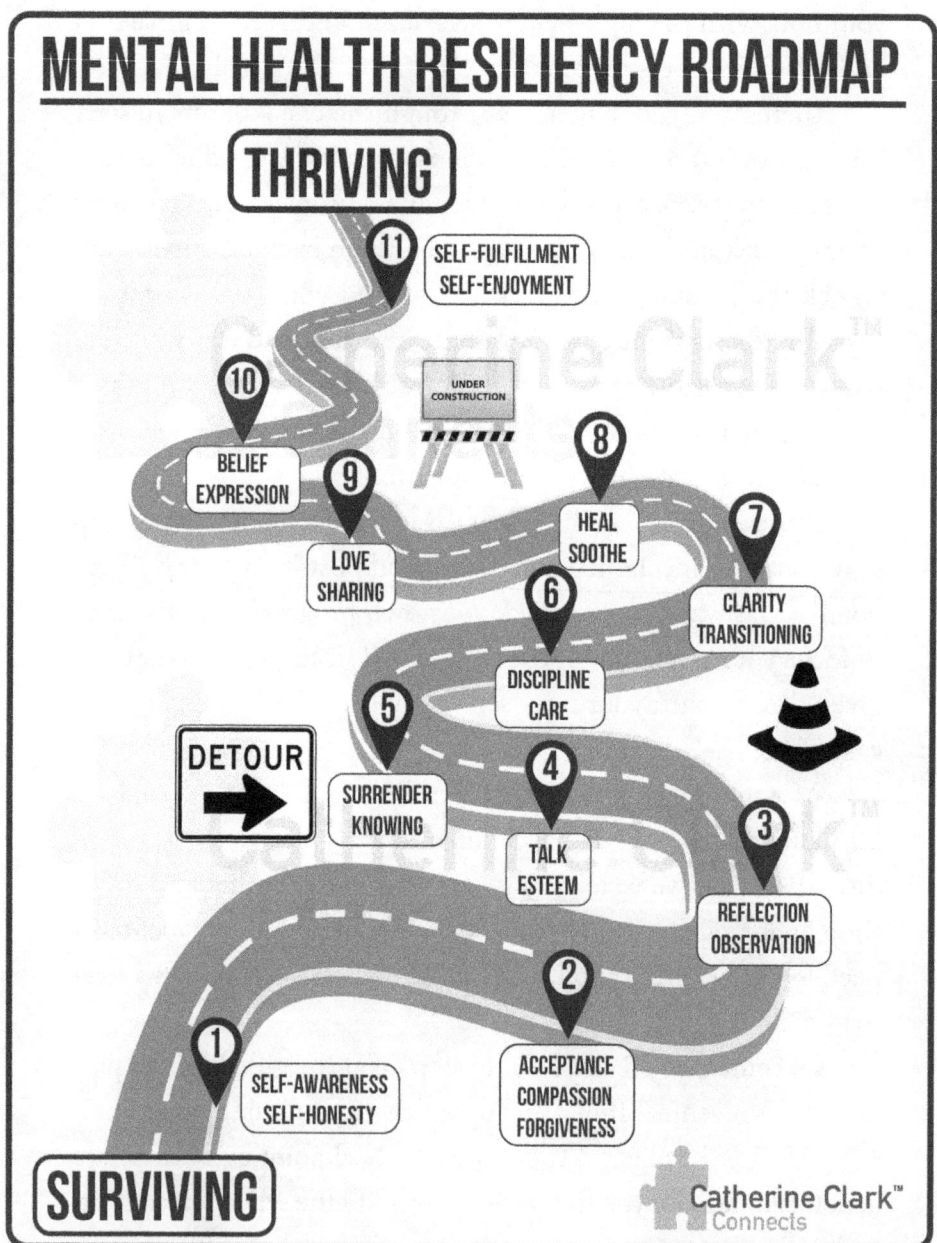

It might also be helpful to start a mental health resiliency travel journal to record action items, thoughts and insights that arise throughout your journey. You can also use the blank pages at the back of the book to jot down your notes. Better yet, be unorthodox and write all over the pages — highlight, earmark, scribble, rip out pages — and surrender to whatever process is motivating and empowering for you. Read, rest, digest and track your progress on the roadmap for even deeper insights into your dark gifts.

Please don't focus too much on the destination, but rather enjoy the ride and embrace the journey toward self-enjoyment. Creating lasting change is about making small yet significant course corrections, telling yourself the truth, being patient in "construction zones," taking detours when needed, learning, growing, finding micro-moments of joy and unwrapping your dark gifts as you collect resiliency tools along the roadway.

PART ONE

ACKNOWLEDGE YOUR GIFTS IN DARK PACKAGES

CHECKPOINT 1

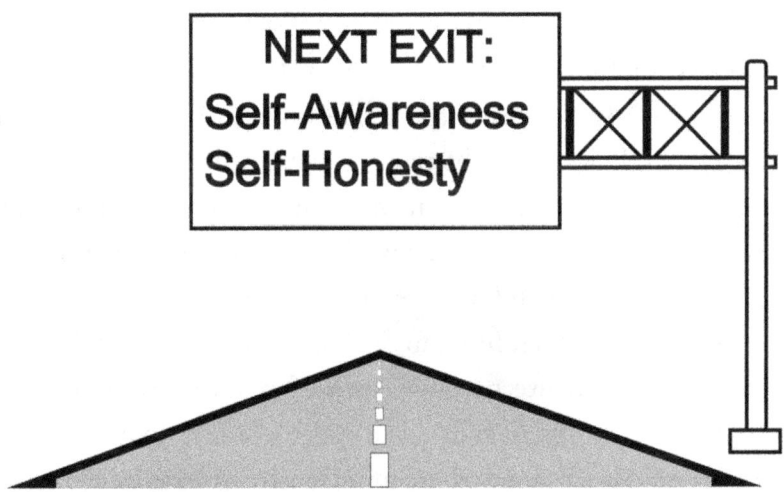

"Until we have met the monsters in ourselves, we keep trying to slay them in the outer world. And we find that we cannot. For all darkness in the world stems from darkness in the heart. And it is there that we must do our work."
— Marianne Williamson

HOTEL SASKATCHEWAN BREAKDOWN

I fell up the grand staircase of the historic Hotel Saskatchewan. Yes, up!

I was a complete mess juxtaposed against the majesty of red-carpeted stairs and shiny brass railings that have welcomed white-gloved Queens since the 1920s. There was no hiding my fall and it was in no way regal. It was the kind of wipeout usually only witnessed on the ski hill. Pumpkin spice latte dripped from my wannabe boss-lady trench coat as I watched my life splatter before me in slow motion, ugly brown droplets. I was paralyzed.

"Is this it? The complete, all-out breaking point?" I asked myself. My peripheral vision caught sight of a stately bellboy's hand as I was helped to my feet. At that moment, I responded internally, "No, not yet. I'm finishing this workshop, dammit, but I'll book my nervous breakdown for November 1, 2019."

Ironically, I'd been hired to facilitate a full-day mental health training session with executives who needed to learn how to recognize the signs of mental illness and build a bridge to access timely resources and support. My job was to share my extensive knowledge of mental health and teach communication techniques so managers could effectively intervene and prevent stressed-out, overwhelmed employees from having a full-blown mental breakdown.

I believe I stopped just short of saying, "This session is brought to you today by a mental health professional on the brink of a nervous breakdown!"

One thing that happens when you're on the verge of a breakdown — you get very, very real. The raw, authentic type of real where you don't have an ounce of energy left to care about wordsmithing or what people think. I'm pretty sure that I spoke of being in the midst of a devastating marital separation, suicidal ideation and my raw trauma work in the Arctic where the suicide rate is ten times the national average. The most surprising thing of all was that they loved my facilitation style. I'll never know for sure what I said but I was personally requested as a preferred facilitator by that company thereafter.

I learned something about resiliency that day, something I had never fully put into practice in all my years of counselling and training. Our true superpower and strength are our self-honesty and vulnerability. It's having self-awareness and presence of mind to know when you're in over your head — completely overwhelmed — and when you need to ask for help. These are the things we will learn at this first highway exit.

But knowing when you're psychologically drowning isn't something we're taught or socialized to acknowledge, is it?

The thing is, most of us don't have a mental health gauge at all. We just keep pushing and numbing our unconscious thoughts until we finally collapse. It's often a painfully slow erosion of mind, body and spirit, so no one even notices.

They see the hustle.

They see the energizer bunny.

Then the battery just fizzles out and we fall off the map.

Yes, a trained professional is just as likely as anyone else to ignore signs of burnout and fall flat on her face — maybe even more so.

That's why we need mental health resiliency — a set of informed wellness practices — physical, cognitive, emotional and spiritual that empower you to withstand and learn from difficult and traumatic experiences. These practices will help you move through any adversity to arrive at the next best version of yourself.

When you deny the dark story in your past, it defines and limits the ability of your future self to thrive. It can keep you stuck in a downward spiral of victimhood, fear and shame. But when you own your dark story, it informs you, builds inner confidence and propels you into uncharted waters. You can sail a whole new ship and write a brand new life chapter.

Believe me, this approach is so much better than repeating the same behaviors with the same adverse repercussions. Life will keep throwing us challenges — that's for sure. We can't stop dark packages or difficult experiences from coming. The difference is learning how to acknowledge and fully experience adversity — viewing it as an opportunity to fine-tune your inner powers — a chance to find the meaning in your mess.

So, how do you even start to acknowledge messy emotions?

Dr. Paul Ekman, a leading expert on emotions, identified that there are seven universal emotions and accompanying facial expressions that exist across all cultures: anger, fear, joy, surprise, sadness, disgust and contempt.[1] Although there are differing views among experts, most emotion scientists agree on these core emotions. Within each of these central themes, we have thousands of sub-emotions and feelings. It's like we have a super-advanced "feelings information dashboard" at the ready. Yet most of the time, the emotional responses that shape our experiences are completely unconscious.

In her recent book, *Atlas of the Heart*, Brené Brown has taken emotion research to new heights, uncovering and bringing to light eighty-seven distinct human emotions. Her central premise is contrasting and distinguishing similar, conflated or confusing emotions — such as shame and guilt — and discussing ways to navigate these emotions for ourselves and others.[2] This challenge reinforces the importance of understanding and naming our feelings as one of the first steps to safely processing adversity and healing our pain.

So, at this first checkpoint, you'll need to lift the lid and look under the hood of your car. Maybe you'll be shocked by what you find — maybe you won't. Either way, you can start to acknowledge all the parts of you — weak, loving, overzealous, ashamed, spiteful — you've kept hidden in a dark box with that gold star and shiny veneer. You can finally move beyond "barely surviving" and get back on the road to "thriving."

FEELING IS HEALING

The very first tool you'll need on this journey is an effective way to process intense emotional experiences — to recognize emotions that arise — as you hold your dark package in your hands. Scary, I know. It's natural to want to avoid your feelings, especially those linked to an unpleasant experience. Most of us would rather ignore these signals — the warning signs that we're on the verge of a breakdown — until the eleventh hour. I'm guilty, as charged. If we ignore our feelings, we stay entrenched in them — then we end up yelling at the barista who messed up our half sweet, skim, no whip, cinnamon dolce latte, or we engage in road rage with a granny in a school zone.

Yes, we can unlearn this auto-pilot response, become more self-aware and "feel it all to heal it all." When we call out our fear, we can see it as separate from who we really are. Then we're able to observe our experience from a distance with a more open heart, and that's when we can start to breathe a huge sigh of relief.

But I'd rather run and hide too. I did it for years.

Yet, we need our emotions. They're there for good reason. They keep us safe and have real survival value. Emotions are governed by the limbic system in our brain — our gut reactions to any situation. The kingpin of this information system is the amygdala, which registers fear and danger. That's what tells us to run for our life when a saber tooth tiger is on the move, or your boss has a pink slip in his hand. It keeps us singing the "Stayin' Alive" song. But if we keep avoiding our emotions or fearful activities like public speaking, our amygdala never learns how to calm down and deactivate the unconscious flight, fight or freeze response.

So, yes, I'm suggesting it's time to tune in, turn up the volume and stop suppressing our feelings — "the messages in the mess." When we suppress the painful emotions, we also suppress the positive emotions — our "super intuition" beacons. That means it's time to stop asking, "Why am I feeling this way?" or saying, "I shouldn't feel this way." Start asking instead, "How does this dark package make me feel?" or, "What is this emotion trying to tell me right now?" Even asking, "What needs to change in my life right now to feel safe, valued and restored in this situation?" is a great question.

There are four main steps to getting our emotional signalling system fired up and roadworthy at this checkpoint.

Step One: Practise Self-Awareness
Turn inward. Visualize your emotions as beautiful messengers trying to gift you with self-insight.

Self-awareness is the art of understanding yourself, fully recognizing what you're feeling, what you're actually experiencing in your body, mind and spirit and taking action. Being quick to anger, feeling on edge or having recurrent gastrointestinal stomach upset are important "information beacons." They're saying, "Hey, please pay attention and help me get through this."

The trick is to stop, get very still, take a deep breath and observe what's happening in your body as an emotion arises. You only need to give yourself thirty seconds to follow your breath all the way in and all the way out a few times. Allow yourself to be completely still — to really notice the wheels turning inside. Then ask, "What do you want me to feel here — what's the message?"

For example, if you're feeling angry that someone may have taken advantage of you, the "feeling messenge" and "gift" in this emotion might be:

Feeling Message: Disrespected or violated.

Gift: I can learn how to set safe boundaries for myself. I can choose only respectful relationships where I feel valued and cared for in the future.

Step Two: Practise Self-Honesty — give yourself permission to authentically "feel"

My personal and professional experience has taught me that when you're painfully honest with yourself, you can be free. There's so much freedom in letting go of the charade. You clear up space to align with good feelings like joy, so you can finally breathe again — phew! Your chances of falling up the stairs on the way to your job also lessen.

In fact, being brutally honest about what you're feeling and giving yourself permission to feel without judgement is a disciplined practice. Feeling your emotions through the lens of self-compassion is the route to uncovering the true "wisdom in your wounds." We'll learn more about self-compassion at Checkpoint 2.

So, for now, whatever you're feeling is perfectly okay. You're not alone. Sometimes, it might feel like you're all alone, and even just being there for yourself can be really hard. Please take all the time you need to just sit in a puddle on the floor if that's where you need to be right now. It's okay to not be okay. Lean into your uncomfortable feelings — envy, shame, bewilderment — whatever they may be. Give yourself the gift of honouring whatever's showing up for you — real, authentic feelings. Give them a voice.

What voice is that, you might ask? Maybe you honestly don't know what or how to feel. That's normal. Processing our emotions is a learned skill — who knew? I would bet it wasn't modelled for you at home growing up. Having worked as a guidance counsellor, I know for certain they don't teach emotional regulation well in school.

Let's face it, most of us have spent our entire lives trying to deny or cover up our feelings. As a child, you may have received programming like: "Don't cry" or "You've got nothing to be angry about." Or your family may have discouraged you from expressing strong emotions of any kind. So, you stopped acknowledging feelings like sadness or anger altogether. Perhaps you grew up in a home where one of your parents would unleash their emotions and hold the rest of the family hostage to them. The unconscious coping strategy you may have picked up and replicated is, "Don't express your feelings or the situation will only escalate."

If you're anything like me, you were told not to be so sensitive, even though you naturally absorb the feelings of everyone else in the room. You had to "keep a lid on it." So, you spent most of your adult life trying not to experience any feelings at all. Or, you may have faced the additional pressure of needing to be super strong — never showing vulnerability or weakness — because that was how you survived and stayed safe. This stoicism is why a close-knit community where you can safely unmask and express your honest feelings is of vital importance. We'll talk more about the importance of a friendship network at Checkpoint 9 and throughout this book.

Step Three: Learn to attach a valid label to what you're feeling — develop a "feeling vocabulary"
Accurately acknowledging and naming our feelings is the next steppingstone to finding relief and mental health resiliency. You might say to yourself, "I feel rejected and irritated when my friend doesn't reply to any of my texts." You're not avoiding or pushing those honest feelings away. In fact, the very act of naming the feeling actually helps reduce its intensity. This naming can make any emotion feel more manageable. It works like a magic eraser for emotional overreaction. It also informs a more adaptive response, such as communicating how you would like to be treated in the future, instead of bottling up your feelings.

A "feeling vocabulary" list such as the following "Emotions Wheel" can make it much easier to unpack and talk about your emotions. Each primary emotion can be broken down into more distinct, nuanced emotions. This activity is a great way to stretch your feelings vocabulary range because as you know, sometimes you just don't know how to feel. That's okay — we're all learning here. Your vocabulary will grow if you regularly practise adding new feeling words to your conversations and interactions.

Of course, the really destabilizing emotions, like shame and grief, can also be the most painful. Understanding these feelings better can help you grow, remain more objective when intense "fight or flight" feelings arise, and learn to be kinder to yourself. Watch for and acknowledge those dark packages when they appear. I recommend you seek out Brené Brown's recent research for some of the best descriptions available for expanding your emotional literacy.

EMOTIONS WHEEL

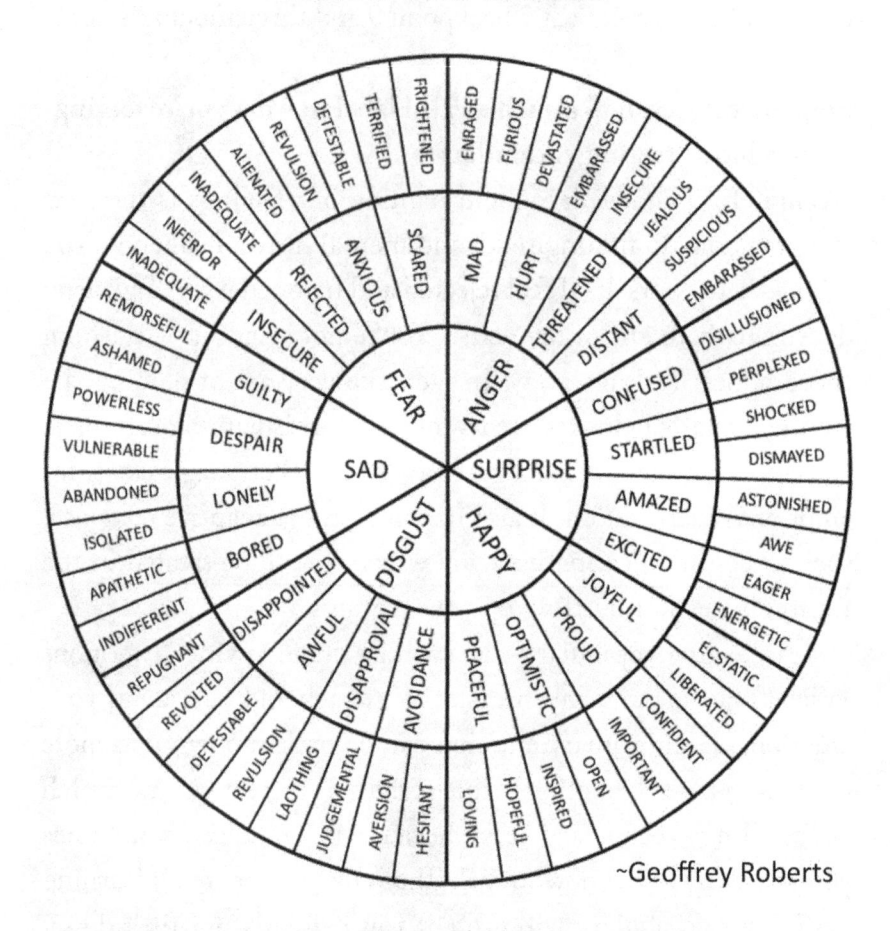

~Geoffrey Roberts

Here's an example of how a "feeling vocabulary" has proven invaluable for healing in my client work:

A couple in their fifties, who had been married for twenty-seven years, had come to see me for relationship counselling. Bitter, resentful and exhausted — they were on the precipice of divorce. Collectively, they wore the look of hopelessness that permeated the room. They'd been stonewalling, undermining and ignoring each other for so long — I seriously wondered if they had any feelings at all.

If you can't label your emotions, then it's nearly impossible to have a collaborative, restorative conversation about how you are feeling. It may sound overly simplistic, but the exercise of merely naming and circling their feelings on a chart together and practising active listening is probably what saved their marriage. The dark gift in their marital breakdown was the opportunity to learn how to wholeheartedly communicate their genuine feelings with one another, to be heard and understood — perhaps for the first time ever.

I've witnessed hundreds of clients bury strong emotions without even realizing what they're doing. Many others use humour to deflect emotions, doing everything possible to laugh away the pain, or mask their emotions with toxic positivity. We'll look more closely at this concept in Part Three.

Just know it's not your fault. We all have trauma — even if you wouldn't call it that — buried somewhere in our psyche. Trauma specialist, Dr. Gabor Maté, author of *When the Body Says No: The Cost of Hidden Stress*, describes childhood trauma as the main cause of repressed emotions — disconnecting from ourselves is a form of numbing and maladaptive coping.[3] It's also one of the key contributing factors to developing a mental disorder such as depression. I often tell my clients that "anger, turned inward" becomes depression. You beat yourself up instead of expressing the anger outwardly. Does this sound familiar? You're not alone — I'm guilty of this too.

Dr. Bessel van der Kolk's book, *The Body Keeps the Score: Brain, Mind and Body in the Healing of Trauma*, is also an amazing resource for anyone who is ready to go deeper in acknowledging their trauma. He describes the first goal of trauma acceptance as making those negative emotions and the accompanying fear more tolerable — to create space for healing.[4]

This trauma-healing approach acknowledges how much your emotions matter. YOU matter. You are a whole person with an immense range of raw, beautiful emotions.

GIFT BOX RESILIENCY TOOLS

Here's how to put this learning to work. Starting today, let's practise self-awareness and self-honesty by learning to acknowledge authentic, "no-holds-barred" feelings. Dig deep and find the part of you that aches in your gut or haunts you when your head hits the pillow at night.

1. **Observational Tool**: Over the course of this week, practise feeling, observing your bodily sensations and experiencing whatever emotion naturally arises, especially strong ones, as you go about your day. Jot down each emotion in your journal. Think of yourself as a researcher collecting data on your authentic experiences and triggers.

2. **Awareness of Feeling Tool**: When you're unable to express a negative feeling, acknowledge that you've been conditioned to override or numb it. Acknowledge and accept the feeling. It has probably been buried and repressed in your dark package. This is a huge step.

> **3. Present Moment Tool**: Feelings come in waves that rise, crest and recede throughout your day. Remind yourself to stop, breathe and simply observe your emotional response with your whole body in the present moment. Neurologists have found that the physiological lifespan of an emotion in the body and brain is only 90 seconds. So, the trick is to not respond immediately or feed a story that keeps you stuck in an emotional loop. Get curious in your observations and laugh at your overreactions. Say to yourself, "This too will pass." By applying this technique, strong emotions like anger, fear, sadness, or shame will start to be less likely to disrupt your life for hours or days as they may have in the past.

The good news is that we can learn to process adversity and acknowledge strong emotions in an adaptive way at any age. It just takes time, patience and practice. The tools you'll pick up at each checkpoint on this road trip will help you continue to do just that.

Luckily, we have the ability to heal ourselves, rise above adversity and learn emotional self-regulation on our own. For some of us, this healing may require medical intervention, the help of a skilled therapist (to work through past trauma) and the support of family/community members. Emotionally focused therapy (EFT) is just one of many therapeutic approaches that may have particular benefit for emotional repression. Another approach, dialectical behavioural therapy (DBT), has been found to be particularly helpful in changing disruptive thought patterns and reframing your story in a more realistic, positive way. But a combination of all modalities — self-help and professional support — tends to be the most healing and restorative approach.

Here's an example of DBT. Take a moment to write down the answers to these prompts and say them out loud:

1. **State a painful past event.** I was severely bullied and ostracized in middle school.

2. **State what caused the event.** I was an artsy, different, painfully shy "new kid" at school. I didn't fit in.

3. **State the feelings.** Abandonment, loneliness, deep sadness and anger at not only the bullies, but all the teachers/adults who did nothing to keep me safe.

4. **State the plan.** These feelings are valid, but they no longer serve me. Now, as an adult, I am choosing to acknowledge all these traumatizing feelings at the bottom of my dark package. I meet the memory of this experience with compassion and can choose to let it go.

Psychologist Brené Brown reinforces this practice by saying, "The most powerful moments of our lives happen when we string together the small flickers of light created by courage, compassion and connection and see them shine in the darkness of our struggles."[5] Brown further explains that in order to live a full life, we need to stop avoiding, numbing and dismissing our feelings and instead start to:

- Try on and allow for a full range of emotional experience.
- Observe and become aware of numbing behaviours.
- Learn how to "lean into" and feel uncomfortable, strong, emotions like anger, grief and sadness.

☕ COFFEE WITH CATHERINE

Let's say we have stopped on our road trip for coffee. As we sip our coffee, I'd like you to honestly answer these questions with me:

1. Write down in your journal a hardship or mental health challenge you're currently facing (e.g., breakup, bully boss, ill health, etc.). Ask, "What's really triggering me right now?"
2. Write down the emotions this situation brings up for you.
3. If you feel nothing at all, that's okay. Describe how you might be numbing your feelings (e.g., binge-watching a mini-series, online shopping, emotional eating, gambling, alcohol, etc.).
4. Turn to the Emotions Wheel to come up with a name for your emotional response.
5. Close your eyes, take a deep breath and really tap into the feeling. Say to yourself, "Yes, this is jealousy," or "Yes, this is resentment."

6. What sensations are you experiencing in your body (e.g., chest constriction, back pain, headache) as you name your feelings? Ask yourself, "Where or how am I experiencing this feeling, sensation or pain in my body?" For example, as you're reading this right now you might feel any one of these things: blocked, heaviness or tightness.
7. Tell yourself, "This feeling will pass very quickly." Let it wash over you. Separate the emotion from yourself as if you were observing it in someone else. Reassure yourself that it will dissipate on its own — especially with the help of positive, realistic self-talk that you will learn at Checkpoint 4.
8. Visualize a place where you feel safe, grounded and secure. What are you experiencing in your body now? Observe the change. Breathe. Put this visual image on your bulletin board, screensaver, or bathroom mirror. Transport yourself there any time you are overwhelmed by your feelings.

MAKING MENTAL HEALTH MATTER

> *"Mental health isn't a destination, but a process. It's about the drive, not where you're going or the make of your car."*
> — Catherine Clark

Mental health can be invisible. If I passed you on the street, I'd have no idea what psychological challenges you might be facing. I wouldn't see if there was an imminent breakdown lurking underneath your shiny car. I'd only see your "nice enough" exterior.

The truth is, I've dressed up, put on make-up and shown up for work on time, all the while being completely preoccupied with thoughts of suicide. You can have the biggest smile in the room yet be living with crippling depression on the inside.

Since this journey will be a long road trip, let's do a mental health safety check to make sure your vehicle is completely roadworthy. Yes, I can see you squirming in your seat. It's okay. We just have to look under the hood again, change a few psychological filters, maybe even get some new spark plugs. We just did an emotional (feelings) check-in, but at this first checkpoint it's also important to take an honest account of your mental health.

Let's face it, at some point in our lives we've all experienced mental health challenges such as: isolation, loneliness, illness or disconnection. Difficult times, like the Covid-19 pandemic, are a catalyst for many mental health issues. Most of us find adaptive ways to cope. For example, avid runners and hikers know that exercise and being in nature elevate your mood — releasing those natural "feel good" endorphins.

But for others, overwhelming emotions can stick around for a long time, interfering with all aspects of our lives, even warranting medical intervention or professional support. Hey, I've been there — it's normal, especially if you have a biochemical or hormonal imbalance. If you've ever experienced a mental health disorder in the past, you know how easy it can be to get mired in self-stigma. Fear and misinformation about mental illness can completely railroad your life, sucking you into a vortex of self-loathing, avoidant behaviour and apathy. Societal stigma prevents many of us from ever accessing services in the first place, to get the help we need.

The good news is that mental health associations across the globe (e.g., Canadian Mental Health Association — CMHA) offer a myriad of free services, such as counselling, psychoeducational resources and psychological assessments.[6] Just reaching out to a friend or calling a mental health helpline can be an important first step on the mental health resiliency roadway.

You can start by using an online tool to help you assess and better gauge your mental health. One of these resources is eMentalHealth.ca which has a range of tools to quickly assess everything from postpartum depression to technology addiction.[7] Therapists, counsellors and medical professionals also have robust inventories to gauge your mental wellness. For example, the Beck Depression Inventory is a questionnaire that I typically use in an initial therapy session to determine whether someone is experiencing temporary blues/depressed mood or meets the criteria for clinical depression.[8]

Suffering poor mental health doesn't mean you're broken, inferior or weak. Mental disorders have no gender, race, socioeconomic status, or face. They are legitimate medical conditions, just like physical illnesses (e.g., cancer or diabetes).

Thank goodness societal stigma is eroding and we're beginning to talk honestly and openly about mental health. You can count me in the statistic that says one in two Canadians will experience a mental disorder before they turn forty.[9] I not only suffered from severe depression but also postpartum depression and generalized anxiety disorder, all before my fortieth birthday. So, you're in good company.

The best news: you can live a happy, healthy, productive life with a mental disorder if you have effective treatment and good coping strategies. Often the most successful treatments are multi-faceted — pharmacological intervention combined with counselling such as cognitive behavioural therapy (CBT) or eye movement desensitization reprogramming (EMDR) and a good exercise program.

Working with courageous clients who are living with mental illness has taught me the power of honesty and authenticity. Pretending to be someone you're not doesn't prevent pain, it increases it. When we hide our truth from others, we suffer deeply. But when we find the strength to confront our emotions and acknowledge a problem, the pain is lessened.

When I suffered my first bout of depression at thirty years old, I thought my life was ruined. In reality, that dark package shaped me into the strong, empathic woman I am today. It's our struggles, past and present, that sow the seeds for authentic growth.

Here's a story of a client who received effective treatment for a mental disorder — emerging from the darkness, fully embodying the learning found within:

I could see the relief wash over Mary's face as she settled into the comfy blue chair and proceeded to tell me that she'd been diagnosed with postpartum depression (PPD). Then she explained how the temporary relief of this diagnosis was quickly overshadowed by feelings of shame. Shame that she couldn't help herself — that she wasn't a competent mother

— started spilling out into the room. She said she felt ashamed that she was even suffering from a mental disorder. I absorbed the gravity of her self-criticism and self-sabotage. I knew it would be a long climb out of this dark hole.

Even with effective interventions like cognitive behavioural therapy and antidepressant medication, it took some time for this workaholic thirty-something career woman to recover from PPD. But, a year later, Mary did make a full recovery. And what did she learn because of this adversity? She found the pathway to being her own best friend. Mary learned that carving out time to pamper herself — enjoying outings on her own — made her a more joyful person and wholehearted, attentive mother. She refashioned her life into something completely different. What would have seemed selfish and indulgent in her past programming was now deemed essential. Mary learned how to love and adore herself first. PPD had given her the gift of self-love — valuing her own time and energy above all else.

I know the feelings of PPD all too well, having experienced it myself after the birth of both of my babies. With each of my pregnancies, I had to advocate for medical intervention because PPD is still highly underdiagnosed and dismissed as postpartum baby blues. Stigma exacerbates silent suffering making it difficult to ask for help.

At this checkpoint, consider, "Where am I on the mental health continuum on a scale from 1 (barely surviving and floundering) to 10 (thriving and flourishing)?"

Can you be honest with yourself today? In what ways might you be struggling? Take a deep breath and write down your number.

Truth be told, are you feeling on the brink of your own Hotel Saskatchewan breakdown? If yes, I'm glad you're here. If you're feeling completely overwhelmed by your inner darkness, please reach out to a loved one, visit a medical practitioner or call a mental health hotline before continuing this journey. I've created a Mental Health Matters resources page on my website at www.catherineclarkconnects.com for specific resources and more detailed information about mental disorders: depression, anxiety and suicide prevention strategies.

So, let's complete this safety check, have another coffee (I do love my coffee) and pick up some tried-and-true mental health strategies at the gift shop.

COFFEE WITH CATHERINE

As we sip our coffee at this rest stop, I'd like you to honestly answer these questions and do these activities:
1. Please share where you're at right now on the mental health scale from 1 (barely surviving) to 10 (optimally thriving). Why do you say that? How will you know when you're thriving? What would you be doing or saying differently then?
2. What would it take to move half a point up on this mental health scale?
3. What's one small step (mental health booster) you could start today? Maybe stop for two minutes to observe your breath, walk in nature, laugh with a friend, reframe a conversation, or eat a healthy snack.
4. Make a list now. Write all possible suggestions down on a paper, cut each suggestion out and place each tiny piece of paper in a "Mental

> Health Booster" jar (use any empty container). Paint or decorate your container so it's uniquely yours. Now you can reach in the jar anytime you need a mental health pick-me-up reminder.

Accept and acknowledge that your mental health needs your loving attention and deserves your support every day. Try these activities over the course of a week and note any improvements in your overall well-being:

1. Write the word "breathe" on a sticky note and put it on your computer. Practise filling your entire belly with air by breathing in through your nose for the count of four, holding for two and then very slowly blowing the air out through your mouth for eight counts, then repeat. This exercise will immediately relieve stress and reduce anxiety.
2. Pick out one mental health booster from your jar twice daily (e.g., take a brisk walk or other form of exercise, play music, call a friend, cuddle your pet, make a healthy meal, etc.).
3. Lifeline list: Write down two personal contacts and two professional contacts on separate sticky notes. Make a duplicate copy. Keep one set in a visible place at your desk. Put the other set in your purse or wallet. Now you have a handy "who you gonna call?" list for when the shit hits the fan and the Ghostbusters aren't answering.
4. Call each person on your lifeline list (or leave a voice memo) to let them know how important they are to you today.

REDISCOVERING YOUR RESILIENT HERO

"Hard times don't create heroes. It is during the hard times when the 'hero' within us is revealed."
— Bob Riley

There's a reason why the rear-view mirror in our car is so small in comparison to the windshield. Both are important. We can't ignore what's behind us — what made us the resilient hero we are today. But, if we're fixated on the past, or if we completely avoid our dark stories, we can stay stuck in that rear view. We cannot see the wide-angle view of the windshield — the landscape of immense possibilities that lie ahead — unless we acknowledge what is within.

So, at this checkpoint let's also validate and honour how resilient you already are — what you've survived. Look at the trials and tribulations you've faced — the dark packages — even if they do not seem like capital "T" traumas. There's growth to be found in all of our challenges that enables us to move through them and find the gift of transformation that our souls are seeking.

Please take a moment now to consider what would be the most debilitating yet transformative dark package you've ever been handed. I mean the one that actually changed your life for the better — made you feel like a resilient hero. Jot it down in your journal if it's safe to do so.

I'd like to share with you a doozy of a story — one of my darkest packages. Even if you're a professional therapist, you can't necessarily avoid damaging relationships. None of us can. In fact, my own life has been just as messy as the lives of my clients. You see, being a counsellor doesn't suddenly make you immune from life's lessons. All these "gifts" that I've learned personally have only enhanced my professional skills. There is real value in life experience and overcoming obstacles that simply cannot be taught. Staring fear down and owning our resilient spirit is our number one priority.

Here's one of the dark packages that I was handed more than thirty years ago. I was twenty-eight years old, and on marriage number one:

I wondered to myself, "How could things have gone so terribly wrong?" The couples' psychologist said our relationship had been based on what he called the Hollywood romance model. In effect, my husband was all about the conquest. It's not a new story and surely it is one of the classic Hollywood movie plot lines. The whole thrill of the chase was what I understood to be the premise of my husband's desire. I, on the other hand, had entered the institution of marriage with the old-fashioned idea that people honour and respect one another, are faithful and stay together for a lifetime once they have found "the one." Yes, that's the classic, "happily ever after," white wedding, conditioned ideal.

Even though I suspected it, the moment I found the evidence, my heart sank with the grim reality I had feared all along: my husband is having an affair. Graver yet, we'd barely had our first anniversary. If it had been one lapse in judgement — one night of wild abandonment — there might have been hope for repairing fractured trust.

But things only got worse and more sinister from there. The sneaking around, the lying and money disappearing all continued, and the psychological abuse escalated. Insidious gaslighting soon took me down a pathway of self-doubt and self-abandonment. When you're separated from your family and closest friends, it's easy to lose track of your own values and self-worth. You feel fractured and torn apart by the one person who is supposed to love you more than anyone else on this earth.

Still, I remained silent, questioning my own culpability and morals. Then I finally spoke up — threatened to leave. And so it began all over again — the "I'm sorry," "I'll stop," roses-and-chocolates honeymoon phase. This is a classic cycle of abuse, but with a narcissistic twist that oddly enough leaves you, the victim, feeling responsible for the marital breakdown, while the abuser seems faultless.

I finally confronted him with evidence of his cheating, lying, sexual promiscuity and high-risk behaviour. His hollow, unflustered response to this confrontation spoke volumes. He was not remorseful in any way. My marriage was over. Like so many others in abusive relationships, you almost need the jaws of life to extract yourself from the carnage.

It's worth repeating: the best resiliency lessons and blessings are found in the darkest boxes. So, after unpacking and processing the emotional horror that was my first marriage, what did I learn?

Dark Package: Infidelity and relationship breakdown
Message: Disrespect, self-abandonment and self-betrayal
The Gift: I learned to stop having intimate relationships that I did not choose, but where I was chosen. I learned to stand in self-love, first and foremost, and choose partners who are worthy of my time, energy and love. I also discovered the joys and freedoms of being self-partnered. We will do a deeper dive into these practices at Checkpoint 9.

Being a resilient hero means you get back up. You live. You learn. You slay your dragons. What choice do you have when you're literally sideswiped by a dark package?

I'm sure you have a similar story when you were betrayed, abandoned, or kicked to the curb. Yet, somehow, you mustered up the strength to get back on the road to a better life than the one before. Or maybe you're still feeling stuck in that pain right now?

That's okay. I'm here to remind you that you've survived one hundred per cent of all your very worst days. You're still here. Those searing hardships, like abusive relationships, are the gifts that propel our lives forward in a whole new direction. They remind us that we're the resilient hero of our own life story.

I'd suggest you take an honest, detailed account of your dark packages (writing a timeline in your journal, with specific dates of difficult or traumatic events) so you can finally fully acknowledge all that you've survived. Wow. Take all the time you need to ponder and complete this illuminating exercise.

Here's another example of how fully acknowledging your dark packages can rewrite your hero story and get you back on track on the Mental Health Resiliency Roadmap:

Steve, a client in his mid-forties, came to therapy after having experienced failed relationship after failed relationship. It was clear that he suffered from a crippling fear of abandonment and attachment issues. During therapy, he was able to identify, unpack, fully acknowledge and experience (for the first time) feelings of anger and mistrust after being left at the altar in his late twenties by his high school sweetheart. Only then was he able to release the grip of this profound grief and "loser" story that held him captive — stifling his ability to give and receive love. Steve was finally able to author a whole new "self-love" story so that he could fully open up to the secure love of a worthy partner.

Your soul recognizes and knows your truth. This first checkpoint has been about telling yourself this truth, if you can muster up the courage to do so, to write it all down and tell a professional or trustworthy person your painful story. It's liberating. After doing this exercise, I recommend that you tell that story over and over again until it loses its power over you. Quite simply you won't need to tell your story anymore. And you'll be well on your way to mental health resiliency.

You are already a hero and "more than enough." You have resiliency deep within your bones, and there's no time like the present to lift the lid and bring it all up to the surface. Let's stop chasing "enough" and finally accept that we have all that we need to thrive on this quest. At Checkpoint 2, we'll gather up a set of even more focused tools to do just that. But for now, I invite you to channel your resilient hero so you'll be ready to spring into action whenever the next life tsunami strikes.

Let's top up that coffee and have one last chat at this rest stop.

☕ COFFEE WITH CATHERINE

1. If you could be any superhero, who would you pick?
2. How would you describe your superhero resiliency superpower?
3. Tell me about a time when you tapped this superpower to tackle a mental health challenge or difficult life situation?
4. How did your superpower help you get through this adversity? What helped you cope? How might it help you in the future? What would you do differently next time?

PONDERING POST-TRAUMATIC GROWTH

> *"The wound is the place where the light enters you."*
> — Rumi

As we drive our "resilient hero" cars toward Checkpoint 2, let's also acknowledge that dark gifts help us evolve, thrive and foster what is known as post-traumatic growth (PTG). PTG is a fancy term for a phenomenon psychologists have been studying over the past twenty-five years. Researchers have found that negative experiences really can result in positive change, including newfound personal strengths, improved relationships, a deeper appreciation for life, spiritual growth and exploration of new possibilities.[10] Many people have found that they experience a stronger sense of self as a result of having endured a period of great adversity or chaos. This experience has been called "the dark night of the soul," a term rooted in medieval Christianity used to describe the mental breakdown that many mystics experienced prior to a spiritual awakening.

On this road trip we'll just keep calling our adversities "dark packages" — job loss, economic stress, serious illness, bereavement, relationship breakdown, depression and isolation — the catalysts for discovering a whole new way of being.

Let's also challenge the adage of, "What doesn't kill you makes you stronger and better." Then, everyone who's ever been traumatized would be flourishing and living a great life already — right? The reality is that adversity creates an opening — a moment in our lives. It can bury us in crippling pain or provide an opportunity for painful growth. As children we did not have competencies or coping tools other than maladaptive coping mechanisms like "numbing." Ultimately, as adults, we can choose how to apply our minds, our spirits and reach out for community or cultural resources that support healing and growth, or not. It's worth repeating — we can stay stuck, pretending a dark package doesn't even belong to us, or receive it with open arms, pack it in our car and see where the journey takes us.

There's an interesting study about PTG that was published in the *British Journal of Psychiatry* during the Covid-19 pandemic. It looked at the attitudes of caregivers of children aged six to sixteen who had experienced considerable adversity during the pandemic. But when asked, "Do you think there are any positives coming out of the pandemic?" eighty percent of respondents answered a resounding "yes!" Most described the growth in their family/interpersonal relationships, a greater appreciation for the fragility of life, the need to set new priorities for work-life integration and to build a stronger spiritual base and sense of community.[11]

So, PTG is the dark gift — the struggle to reconstruct our lives after our worldview and conditioned beliefs have been shattered. This dark gift can lead to shifting priorities and pivotal changes that may greatly benefit both your life and the lives of many others.

One example is Candace Lightner, who founded Mothers Against Drunk Driving (MADD) in 1980 after her thirteen-year-old daughter, Cari, was killed by a drunk driver. According to their website, since 1980 MADD reports that they have helped to cut drunk driving deaths in half, saved around 350,000 lives and helped more than 850,000 victims to cope with loss.[12] Dark gifts can motivate us to make a highly positive impact on the world.

Post-traumatic growth is probably what helped you bounce back from your last traumatic experience — no matter how big or small. And it's the gift to be opened in your current life challenge.

Here's a good example of post-traumatic growth of a client that I'll call Ruth. She experienced PTG when she could finally acknowledge the depths of her dark package, and save herself and her children from an abusive relationship.

When Ruth came to my office for the first time, she was distraught. She had struggled with raising two small children within the confines of an abusive relationship for more than seven years. Not surprisingly, she'd grown up in a household with a narcissistic, alcoholic father. Therefore, her tumultuous, life-fearing marriage felt eerily familiar and somehow that it was "what she deserved." After several therapy sessions (with a nailed down safety plan in tow), Ruth was ready to risk ending her marriage. She was able to acknowledge the extent of her self-abandonment and that she had no agency. She was finally ready to escape — ready to leave the relationship and metaphorically jump in the unknown rapids — if not for herself, then for the sake of her children. This courageous action, this moment of unbridled trust in a better future, led her to experience the depth of her own powerful truth — she did, indeed, have agency, freedom and control over her future.

In a follow-up session, she described her metaphorical leap into the unknown (post-traumatic growth) as follows:

"I didn't believe I could swim, and I thought I'd drown in the rapids on my own. But then I found my stroke and got to the other side of that churning river with a newfound sense of strength and self-confidence that I never would have otherwise known!"

Ruth told me she never imagined her life could be so much lighter and easier once she'd freed herself from the chains of such a controlling, unhealthy relationship.

Let's examine PTG by picking up one last resiliency tool from the gift shop before getting back on the road.

GIFT BOX RESILIENCY TOOLS

Here are three simple steps to uncover your own post-traumatic growth:

Step 1: You can get started by naming, writing down or speaking out loud about a specific adversity — dark package — in your life. You can use the same event as before if you like.

Step 2: Say "thank you" for the feelings this adversity triggers, like jealousy, sadness or shame. Turn to your handy Emotions Wheel so that you can label the full range of your emotional experience. Remember to acknowledge your feelings by stating them matter-of-factly like, "This is guilt," or "This is shame."

Step 3: Ask, "How has this dark package motivated me to change my behaviour and evolve for the better? How am I serving my highest good or helping others? Or am I still stuck in this pain and trauma?" Ask a good friend or family member if they have noticed a transformation in you or a change for the better. We will revisit this question at Checkpoint 11.

PART TWO

ACCEPT

YOUR GIFTS IN DARK PACKAGES

CHECKPOINT 2

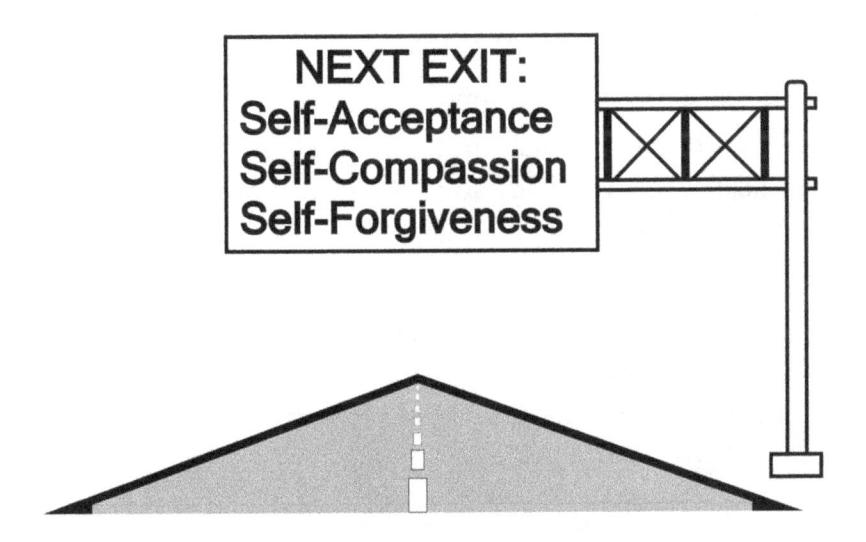

NEXT EXIT:
Self-Acceptance
Self-Compassion
Self-Forgiveness

"I was once afraid of people saying, 'Who does she think she is?' Now I have the courage to stand and say, 'This is who I am.'"
— Oprah Winfrey

For more than two decades, I've answered urgent calls, conducted critical incident stress debriefing for bank robbery victims, held space in talking circles with mothers who have lost a child, and helped managers and employees learn to trust one another after a violent workplace incident. In each of these worst-case scenarios, people respond in one of two ways: either they are completely stopped in their tracks by fear and loss, or they stare down fear and are somehow able to embrace the trauma. Both are normal responses to a traumatic event.

When sideswiped by a terrible incident, you may experience a wide range of physical, emotional and spiritual reactions. These include short-term shock, denial and broken trust, as well as longer-term headaches, gastrointestinal upset and even nightmarish flashbacks. It's completely normal to feel like your sense of safety — what you have known to be true — has unravelled.

Accepting and embracing the experience of being unhinged is not something we're encouraged to do.

Let's face it, if someone said, "Here's your dark package to hold in your hands and make you feel like absolute crap," you'd say, "No way, send it back!"

The thing is, there's no going back. The tide has turned and you've been swept ashore. Maybe it's time to just surrender — have compassion for yourself — relinquish control and ask for help.

Easier said than done, I know.

But that's the only way you can hear the whispers echoing in your dark box — whether you're ready to hear them, or not. With time, you'll look back and see the powerful insights that can come from accepting your dark package. Acceptance requires the necessary ingredients of self-compassion and self-forgiveness. So, you'll want to pick up those traits at this checkpoint to move forward.

ACCEPT YOUR GIFTS IN DARK PACKAGES

Like many of my clients — when I was on the brink of overwhelming trauma with dark packages at my doorstep — moving forward wasn't something that I could just do. I had to completely relinquish control to get unstuck and embrace the necessary reinforcements on the road to self-acceptance.

At the age of thirty, I found myself teetering on the edge of a subway platform. It wasn't pretty. I had no idea that I was suffering from major depression. It was as though a dark freight train had crashed in my brain and knocked out all the power. I was overwhelmed. I just needed to get off the emotional train wreck and escape all the pain — just end it.

I am grateful that my best friend understood suicidal ideation and drove through the night to get me the medical intervention that I desperately needed. The long climb out of this dark hole was an arduous process. But with antidepressant medication that rebooted my biochemistry, and cognitive behavioural therapy to tackle my self-sabotaging thoughts, my depression started to lift.

It was almost as though I'd been given the freedom to climb inside my box of darkness, bitterness and grief — permission to find a whole new sense of self. And that's when I could start edging along the pathway toward self-acceptance.

Of course, as human beings we innately move toward pleasure and away from pain. We want to avoid the shadows of the past — terrible events we survived — at any cost. Who wouldn't? We don't want to get quiet — let thoughts creep in. The last thing we're prepared to do is look into the deep end of our life with compassion and forgiveness.

Yet because you picked up this book, I have every confidence you're ready to at least dangle your feet in the shallow end of self-acceptance. You can keep running forever or you can swim down to the bottom of your dark lake to retrieve the parts you've abandoned. The parts of yourself you've disowned — the battered, broken, joyless parts — the unresolved big "T" and little "t" traumas. Maybe you're in a place where you only want to dip your toe in the water, or maybe you're ready to deep-dive into your murky lake. Wherever you are, it's okay — you can navigate this journey at your own pace.

Up until now, those abandoned parts of you have been floundering in your psyche, waiting to be welcomed in. Perhaps the chaos had to settle, the fog had to lift, for you to finally embrace your shadow self. Now, as a wiser adult, I'd like to suggest you greet those abandoned beings. Hug them like crazy and invite them to be part of your new, mentally healthy narrative. Picture yourself rising from that murky bottom, giving your new integrated self a giant high five.

Because it's finally time to be your own best friend and embrace all of YOU. After all, the longest relationship you'll ever have is the one with yourself.

In Part One, you were encouraged to acknowledge your messy emotions, practise self-awareness, stretch your feeling vocabulary and evaluate your mental health status. You learned to step back, reflect and observe your experience from a safe distance — as a resilient hero. It's easier to do as an adult because you have the reasoning ability, coping tools and choices you didn't have when you were younger. Marvel at how you survived each of those difficult moments when you thought you might not. But you did, and you've kept on surviving. How amazing is that?

In Part Two of this road trip, I encourage you to practise self-acceptance, self-compassion and self-forgiveness — critical ingredients for finding the light in your dark story. Let's walk through the next few exercises together with gentleness and curiosity.

ACCEPT YOUR GIFTS IN DARK PACKAGES   57

For those of you who are currently living with a mental health challenge — depressed mood, anxiety or addiction, for instance — accepting your shadow self, albeit painful, comes with undeniably positive benefits. That being said, reaching out to a trained therapist or close, empathic friend may be a necessary and supportive way to continue on this self-discovery road trip.

First, let's clarify what we mean by these concepts:

1. **Self-Acceptance**: A feeling of satisfaction with yourself, your strengths, talents, body and self-worth — despite any perceived inadequacies, past mistakes and imperfections. Carl Jung described this feeling as embracing your dark side or "shadow self," which I refer to as your "dark package" or "dark story."

2. **Self-Compassion**: A practice of goodwill toward yourself, not necessarily just having good feelings. With self-compassion, we mindfully accept that the moment is painful and embrace ourselves with kindness and care in response, remembering that imperfection is part of the shared human experience — "common humanity." Christopher Germer, a leading compassion researcher, describes self-compassion as, "Simply giving the same kindness to ourselves that we would give to others."[13]

3. **Self-Forgiveness**: Withholding judgement and allowing yourself to move forward without the heavy burden of hanging on to all the mistakes of the past, and instead trying to look at your mistakes as gifts.

Did you know when you can forgive yourself for past failures and love yourself unconditionally, you feel less anxious, angry and sad? If you have self-compassion, you can literally rewire and activate the neurotransmitters in the pleasure center of your brain. Isn't that a good reason to add this trait to your resiliency toolkit? And wouldn't it also be a huge relief to have self-acceptance, "to fully embrace who you are without all the qualifications, conditions, or exceptions"[14]? To me, self-acceptance is being able to say, "I'm enough," and, "I'm worthy of love and respect despite my past mistakes." It's the superhighway to greater joy, self-esteem, recovery and well-being. So, let's not miss all the good stuff at this exit.

First, I want to come clean with you. Although I often teach and encourage each of these practices, I have failed miserably at all of them in the past.

The thing is, I've had to work really hard to counteract imposter syndrome in my many endeavours and to focus on the positive instead of automatically defaulting to the negative. Are you with me on this one? It's like you're all dressed up and rockin' self-confidence until that one uninvited guest makes an off-handed remark. Then it all unravels — and you're suddenly exposed in all your "not good enoughs."

This negative self-talk is why we must flex our acceptance, compassion and forgiveness muscles, which sometimes means getting out of our own way.

To paraphrase a key principle from Eckhart Tolle's renowned book, *The Power of Now*, you simply need to breathe, observe yourself in this moment, acknowledge that the protective shell of your egoic mind is making up a self-limiting story about you, lay down your weapons and create space for a new sense of self to emerge.[15] Woah, that's a mouthful! Yet, I'm confident we can do this together. At the next few checkpoints, we'll add additional tools like mindfulness and cognitive behavioural strategies to make it all come together. But for now, let's delve deeper into self-acceptance.

ALIGNING WITH SELF-ACCEPTANCE

> *"Radical acceptance is the willingness to experience ourselves and our life as it is. A moment of radical acceptance is a moment of genuine freedom."*
> — Tara Brach

We have a human tendency to set rigid high expectations for ourselves. I'd like to offer the liberating idea that you don't have to try so hard to get things right — to achieve some societal standard of perfection — in order to love and accept yourself. After so many years of struggling alongside my clients with the "never good enough" mindset, I've finally stepped off that dance floor.

I've found a whole new break-free dance that's all mine, and you can too. I'm no longer engaging in conversations like the one I've had multiple times throughout my life with my wonderful mother. In a recent exchange, my deep desire for unconditional self-acceptance was reignited. I was trying to articulate how I could be very happy in my life without a husband or the white picket fence programming of the fifties generation. Here's how the conversation went:

"When are you ever going to just settle down?" my Mom asked for the gazillionth time.

"How about never, Mom!" a voice emerged from the darkest depths of my blocked inner child, a place buried so deep in "not good enoughs," I can still feel waves of inferiority reverberating throughout the room.

"Why would I ever want to settle for a so-called comfortable life where a little part of me dies every day? Or accept a state of being where I stop risking, give up on my own dreams and sacrifice my time and energy in a never-ending cycle of serving others?"

"Been there, done that!" I exclaimed.

"Well, if you'd only married the right husband, you'd know how great it is to settle down with your true love and live a happy life," my Mom retorted.

As Glennon Doyle acknowledges in her book, *Untamed*, I lost some of my spark — the raw "me" — at about ten years of age.[16] At this age, I internalized what "good girls" need to do in this world to be liked, and to survive. Also, I was told you don't order Coquilles St. Jacques in a steak restaurant. If you want to get an "A" you'd better colour inside the lines. "Don't be so difficult," "Don't make waves," "You're being way too sensitive and emotional," and, "Why don't you act more like that choir girl at Sunday School?"

These beliefs get ingrained in your programming and dim your light. At this age, you start to settle for what girls of my generation were socialized to be — obedient, watered down, people-pleasers. No mention of thriving, just surviving. Accept the "that's just the way life is" messaging. Where's the freedom of expression and self-acceptance in that? Thank goodness my Gen Z daughter is radically rejecting this programming today.

Many of us are born into families with a cultural worldview that values status, competition and conformity. We learn very early on how to meet the unrealistic expectations of others, while negating our own needs and voice. It's flawed programming — holding yourself to an impossibly high standard while overlooking your actual admirable traits and accomplishments. So, we learn to be experts at focusing on our failures and discounting the positives.

This programming makes it hard to embrace the beautiful, flawed creatures that we are, loving and accepting all our parts: the good, the bad, even the ugly. Wildly and unapologetically, enthusiastically and powerfully, let's walk away from people-pleasing and self-sabotaging. Let's embrace a whole new landscape and get on the road to unconditional self-acceptance. For me, that means being ready to live my soul's purpose and fully embracing my authentic self. A captivating and extraordinary me, scarred from head to toe by so many surgeries that I've lost count!

So, after way too many decades of "not good enough" programming, how can we possibly do that? Let's stop for coffee and ponder that question.

☕ COFFEE WITH CATHERINE

Question:
If you could write a letter of self-acceptance from the perspective of your wise ninety-year-old self to the person you are now, what would you say? What wisdom would you share?

Answer:
What would I tell the younger me who was so depressed and avoidant of the dark gifts in her thirties? What would I tell the sixty-year-old wise woman in me who continues to suffer at the hands of narcissists and reverberates with the sting of self-abandonment and self-criticism? I'd say, "I love you unconditionally. You're very courageous, strong

and resilient. Yes, your depression has marked and defined difficult times in your life, but it doesn't define you."

I would say, "Look at what you've learned from all of your deep dark experiences — look at how you've grown into self-acceptance and embraced your many flaws." I'd highlight the beautiful scars I've collected from head to toe as a record of all my misfortune — a record of living out loud — a testament to riveting risk-taking. The ninety-year-old wise woman in me would celebrate both the visible and invisible scars as the most valuable teachable moments throughout my life.

The wise woman in me would say, "Thank you, body, mind and spirit, for carrying the burden of responsibility for ancestral trauma (the pain and grief of past generations)." She'd thank me for artfully using my words and voice for inner healing and helping others to rise above their own adversity. My wise woman self would say welcome to a state of pure, unbridled, giddy, self-acceptance. The view sure looks great from up here.

What does the wise "elder" in you have for advice? I'm curious.

GIFT BOX RESILIENCY TOOLS

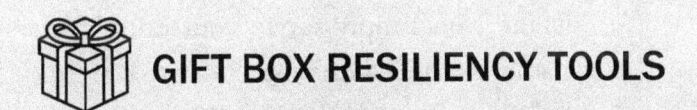

"The curious paradox is that when I accept myself as I am, then I can change."
— Carl Rogers

Self-Acceptance Challenge

Here's a challenge to help you practise self-acceptance today.

Walk into the bathroom or find any mirror. Look straight into your beautiful eyes and say out loud with power in your voice, "I am enough!" and "I love you (insert your name) just the way you are!"

Starting today, repeat these affirmations every morning when you walk into the bathroom and every night before you go to bed for thirty days until you own it and believe it one hundred percent. Observe the transformation in your mindset and self-confidence.

Here are three more of my favourite self-acceptance tools to practise:

1. **Start viewing your failures as interesting happenings.** Pretend you're a researcher collecting data on your day-to-day life. When you make

a mistake, you simply say to yourself, "How fascinating is that? I didn't expect that to happen. I wonder how I could do that differently next time?" This approach helps you reprogram your brain and flips the self-judgement switch off, turning on curiosity and unconditional, positive regard. Neuroscientists call this neuroplasticity, our brain's ability to literally rewire itself and view the world in a new light.

2. **Consider doing a little self-acceptance research project.** Starting today, make a list of every time you notice yourself criticizing or judging yourself harshly. Beside each of these episodes, write down another way to view the situation. What would you say to a friend in a similar situation? With a few tries, you will start to see how your criticism can be shifted to a more realistic, neutral place of self-acceptance.

3. **Stop "playing it safe".** Do you ever make a conscious choice to stay small in your comfortable bubble to avoid humiliation or negative feedback? We all make this choice from time to time to save face. Instead, *try taking little mini risks*, gently nudging yourself toward little mini successes. Like sharing your opinion on a Zoom chat, joining a new

> social club, offering to present a work project or wearing an edgy outfit. I find these small actions can go a long way toward building unconditional self-acceptance. Keep practising!

CREATING SPACE FOR SELF-COMPASSION

Self-criticism and I are very old friends. We've never spent much time apart. My guess is you, too, are beating yourself up right now, dealing with overwhelming regret, fear and an unprecedented level of uncertainty. Then there are those of us who have been raised with the mindset that being hard on yourself is motivating — a good thing. You get more done that way, you achieve more, you never become complacent. This story just makes you feel like crap.

Self-criticism makes you lose faith in yourself and has the opposite effect — you become depressed and unmotivated.

Perhaps you're feeling ashamed of yourself for your latest bad habit, not being a more attentive parent, not focusing on your job, or simply for not being braver. Every single one of us is a direct descendent of ancestors who have survived unthinkable hardships — literally hundreds of generations of survivors. We deserve self-respect for the resourceful, creative, resilient human beings that we are today. It's high time we started serving ourselves compassion instead of relentless self-criticism.

Having courageous, fierce compassion is understanding that so much in life is not your fault, but you are responsible for the way you respond to it.

Self-compassion means choosing love and kindness for yourself and seeing yourself as worthy even when you're feeling broken — *especially* when you're broken — because everyone is worthy of love. In her book, *Fierce Self-Compassion: How Women Can Harness Kindness to Speak Up, Claim Their Power and Thrive*, renowned self-compassion expert, Dr. Kristin Neff, advises women to act courageously in tumultuous times to protect themselves from injustice and abuse, set clear boundaries and celebrate all of their glorious imperfections.[17]

For me, leaving behind a marriage, packing up all my dark packages, squeezing them in my Passat and driving hundreds of miles across the prairies to my new apartment in Toronto constitutes fierce self-compassion. It's giving myself credit for writing a book that has meant painfully reacquainting myself with all the skeletons in my own closet — the parts I've abandoned along the way.

It's channelling bad-ass ferociousness and combining it with tenderness.

It's finding the courage to say "no."

It's saying "no," so you don't lose yourself to the times you said "yes" in the past.

It's finally saying, "Enough suffering already — I deserve to flourish on my own!"

Having compassion for yourself is no different than having compassion for another human being, like the homeless person you pass on the street, as you feel your heartache for them. It's being able to put yourself in their shoes and offer them kindness and understanding, instead of judging them so harshly.

Let's face it, any one of us could be out on the streets — if circumstances were to suddenly change. One of my colleague's clients, a successful retail sales representative for a beverage company became homeless when his only source of revenue — bars and restaurants — closed down in 2020/21 due to Covid-19. This hardship forced him to live out of his car and pitch a tent in the park, unable to pay his rent.

Imagine sending light and love to all beings who are suffering with homelessness right now, through no fault of their own. This compassion for common humanity shows the understanding that suffering is universal for all beings. Compassion literally means "to suffer with" — to walk in another's shoes with a desire to help alleviate their pain.

According to Dr. Neff, "When you feel compassion for another (rather than mere pity), it means that you realize that suffering, failure and imperfection is part of all of our shared human experience."[18] And that helps you connect with a profound sense of suffering in yourself — your own dark story.

This definition of self-compassion has its roots in 2,600-year-old Buddhist writings, but it has since been articulated and refined by Paul Gilbert, the founder of compassion focused therapy (CFT). This form of therapy combines cognitive behavioural therapy (CBT) with neuroscience and Buddhist philosophy. It helps clients connect with their inner wisdom and channel compassion and courage to alleviate suffering from issues like depression, anxiety and PTSD.[19] Dr. Dennis Tirch's, *The Compassionate Mind Guide to Overcoming Anxiety*, is a great place to start if this type of therapy is of interest to you.[20]

The science of compassion is evolving each day as researchers, scientists and thought leaders around the world report "total health" transformations in this field of study. There's a growing body of empirical evidence from biological research and neuroimaging studies that demonstrates how every dimension of our functioning can be enhanced if we exhibit greater levels of compassion. More specifically, self-compassion has been found to positively impact heart rate variability, immune system functioning and our susceptibility to mental illness.[21]

It's easier than you think to start cultivating self-compassion in your life right now. You can start today by simply becoming more conscious of how you talk to yourself.

Here are some ways to get started:

1. Practise speaking to yourself with only kind and loving words for an entire day. That's no small feat. But once you can make it through an entire day, you will feel so much better.
2. Repeat loving affirmations to start your morning and continue throughout the day. You can create a new narrative in your brain's neural pathways with affirmations like: "I am intelligent, creative and abundant." There's a plethora of cell phone apps with affirmations, or you can start by listening on my website: www.catherineclarkconnects.com.
3. Be mindful of stopping the negative descriptors and perfectionistic self-criticism that bubbles up to the surface throughout the day. For example, even saying, "I'm broke," "My financial situation is dire," or, "I'll probably never afford a house," only sets up a scarcity mindset. Saying, "I'm never going to get the job I want," or, "I always mess things up," does not feed self-compassion or self-esteem. Remember that your words have the power to create your reality.

We will focus on challenging and curbing this negative, unrealistic self-talk at Checkpoint 4. But first, we need to build up our self-compassion muscle. How ridiculous is it that we're usually nicer to a complete stranger than we are to ourselves?

So, when self-criticism comes for another visit (as she has every day while I've been writing this book), here's the rebuttal:

Ask yourself, "What would I say to someone else, a friend, or colleague in the exact same situation?"

I know it's an overused cliché but try "being your own best friend." If you're "self-partnered" like me, you truly are the only person who will be there to celebrate your every win and pick up the pieces when you fall up the stairs. Having said that, I have some extra crazy glue and a bottle of Pinot Grigio in my fridge if you need some reinforcements. Let's toast to that: "Goodbye suffering, hello flourishing!"

Now, let's practise our gift box resiliency tools and have a good coffee chat, then I'll tell you some self-forgiveness stories.

🎁 GIFT BOX RESILIENCY TOOLS

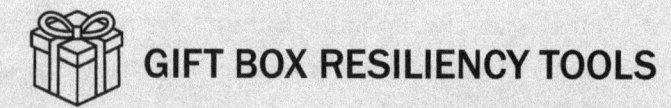

Imagine there's a magical blanket depot you can visit when something traumatic happens in your life. Where you're wrapped up in a super soft blanket of unconditional compassion. It'd be a soothing place where a person with kind, hopeful eyes hands out the blankets and immediately validates your struggle. They would sit with you for as long as it takes for you to let go of self-criticism. There would also be a gentle golden retriever with healing energy cuddled up beside you. You'd feel instantly grounded, loved and grateful.

Wrapped in your blanket, hugging your furry companion, you would finally tap into a spirit of infinite loving kindness for yourself.

This visualization exercise and mental image is something you can bring to mind anytime you need more self-compassion. Give it a try. Is your blanket depot on a calming lake, at the top of a majestic mountain, in the woods, or nestled in a field of daisies?

Let's practise this Self-Compassion Imagery Exercise right now:

- Close your eyes (after you read the instructions) and imagine how it looks, feels, sounds and smells as you wrap yourself in your magical blanket in your favourite place in nature. You can grab a snuggly blanket to use if you like.

- Take a deep breath. Allow yourself to feel the entire scene with all your senses as a white light of unconditional positivity and compassion surrounds you and radiates throughout your whole body.

- Feel the comfort, peace and joy of snuggling up in this soothing blanket of light and self-compassion while repeating these calming words:

"I'm here for you. I love you. Everything will be okay, and I'm never, ever going to abandon you again."

You can repeat this powerful exercise as often as it takes to part ways with your old friend, self-criticism. Cut the cord. Unfriend them now. Move on.

☕ COFFEE WITH CATHERINE

Imagine we're sitting on a comfy couch together, each wrapped in a cozy blanket. You feel warm, safe and supported. I'm in no hurry; I'm here with you. I acknowledge how much you've suffered. I have nothing but love and fierce compassion for you. Take all the time you need to answer these questions:

1. Let's say you wake up tomorrow morning and realise your worst enemy, self-criticism, has finally left for good. What would be the first sign? How would you feel? What would you say or do differently?
2. How will you know when you've completely stopped being so self-critical? What change would you notice in your life, work and relationships?
3. How would your life be transformed once you start hanging out with your new best friend called self-compassion?
4. Do you know someone who needs more self-compassion right now? I suggest you go shopping for a real fuzzy blanket, or better yet, make one — sew, crochet, knit, quilt — with your own two hands. And while you're at it, make or buy one for yourself. Something to always curl up with you, hug you, soothe you and remind you to embrace your gifts in dark packages.

FINDING FREEDOM IN SELF-FORGIVENESS

> *"Darkness cannot drive out darkness; only light can do that.*
> *Hate cannot drive out hate; only love can do that."*
> — Martin Luther King Jr.

In Buddhist philosophy, forgiveness is understood as a way to end suffering — to bring dignity and harmony back to our lives. Forgiveness is fundamentally for our own sake, for our mental health. It's a way to acknowledge and accept the pain we've been carrying around in our dark box — perhaps for years. On the road to self-enjoyment, self-forgiveness is often one of our biggest roadblocks.

Let's face it — we've all been hurt or betrayed by someone before. Knowingly, or unknowingly, we've harmed someone else. We've unfriended someone, lied to a colleague or yelled at our child for singing off-key — killing all their dreams of becoming a pop star. It's inevitable. But we're entitled to stop torturing ourselves about it.

What I've found in my work with clients is that there's a sense of relief to be found in releasing yourself and others from the grip of shame, anger, guilt and resentment that keeps us stuck in suffering. There's freedom on the other side of the "I can't forgive myself" roadblock.

I've witnessed self-forgiveness firsthand in two separate traumatic workplace scenarios. The first situation was a bank robbery where there were employees who could not shake the thought that their actions (or inactions) had caused undue harm to others. The second situation was a workplace construction site accident where negligence played a role in the death of a co-worker. Years later, I met with construction workers who still hadn't forgiven themselves for actions that may have contributed to this lethal accident.

As psychologist Dr. Fred Luskin explains in his book, *Forgive for Good: A Proven Prescription for Health and Happiness*, holding onto guilt, resentment and being unforgiving takes up valuable rental space in your mind leading to chronic negativity, depression and physical illness.[22]

Unfortunately, it's often way easier to forgive someone else than to forgive yourself. Facing the things you don't like about yourself and taking a good hard look at where you made mistakes is really painful. That's where compassion becomes a critical component of forgiveness — acknowledging your own suffering with loving kindness, as well as the suffering you may have caused others. So, if you need to revisit the coffee chat we had on self-compassion just a few pages ago, please do so now.

For those of you who are ready to accept your past transgressions with open arms, I commend you. Your car is going to feel so much lighter as we move forward on this road trip. And don't worry, I'll be practising forgiveness right alongside you. We will gather up tools for self-forgiveness to get unstuck, to forgive yourself for what you didn't know at the time and to move forward.

Phew — what a release! Your tank of gas is going to go much further when you're not so weighed down. Just pull over and toss out that big ugly boulder you've been carting around — that's right, the giant one — the one that's kept you enchained for months, years, or even decades. Let it go.

It never fully belonged to you anyway.

Now put your car in drive and move forward, move beyond and move ahead. The "4 Rs to Forgiveness" will provide you with the resiliency tools you'll need to do just that.

GIFT BOX RESILIENCY TOOLS

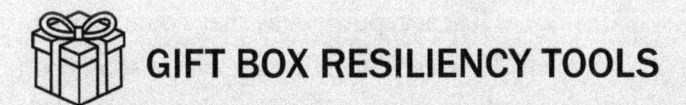

Here's a way to help you start a regular self-forgiveness practice. This tool is critical to your mental health and becoming a road warrior, as the detours, accidents and construction zones continue to show up in your life.

Four Rs to Self-Forgiveness:

1. **RESPONSIBILITY:** Taking an honest account and responsibility for your actions is the first and hardest step. We've all made choices that changed the course of our lives — compromised career, relationships, health and happiness. Realizing that the excuses, rationalizations and justifications are a story you no longer need to tell is the key to moving forward. It's time to fully accept what you have done with complete honesty and self-compassion. I often say to clients, "Tell your story, tell your story, tell your story — until you don't need to tell that story any longer."

2. **REMORSE:** Once you take responsibility for your actions, it's normal to experience remorse and a range of negative emotions. Be still and allow them to wash over you. You may feel guilt

or shame. Just accept them as they come. Say to yourself, "I can still feel like a good person even if I've made a mistake. I'm sorry for my actions. I feel bad about my behaviour and choices, but making a mistake does not make me a bad person."

3. **RESTORATION**: To repair the damage and restore trust, you'll want to apologize, make amends, or take action to rectify your mistakes. It's also the time to say out loud, "I forgive myself." Some of these restorative steps can be very concrete. For example, a partner might make a list of emotional and financial amends that they intend to uphold in a marital separation agreement.

4. **RENEWAL**: What have you learned and how have you grown from this experience? Look for the dark gift. What steps can you take to prevent the same situation from happening again? How can you give back to yourself and others as a result? After my separation, I made a decision to put self-love into practice and leave self-abandonment behind. For me, the dark gift has been spiritual renewal and self-enlightenment.

☕ COFFEE WITH CATHERINE

Let's chat over coffee about other inventive ways to make peace with your dark past and find true self-forgiveness. You could write your own epitaph, summarizing your life by focusing on the things that you are proud of right now (volunteer work, being a good parent, faithful friend, loving spouse, awards, etc). To help you clear any negative energy and remove any blocks, please complete the exercise below:

1. Think of a person in your life who has been like a protector for you, a pet, or an object that makes you feel safe when you wear or hold it (e.g., jewellery, crystal, a letter, etc.). Imagine that you have a safe shield around you with your protector beside you. Take a deep breath.
2. Take responsibility for your faults in an honest way. Say in your mind or write: "I am responsible for _____ and _____ and _____." Let yourself feel it. Breathe.
3. Say to yourself: "But I am not responsible for _____, _____ and _____."
4. Acknowledge what you have already done to learn from your experiences, for reparations and to make amends. Give yourself an appreciative hug.

> 5. Ask if there is anything else that remains to be done and write down how and when you will take this action.
> 6. Finally, say aloud or write: "I forgive myself for _____, _____ and _____." I have taken responsibility for my actions, made amends for what I have done and found a way to make things better.
> 7. Take a deep breath and release. Smile.

FORGIVING OTHERS

> *"Forgiveness is the feeling of peace that emerges as you take your hurt less personally, take responsibility for how you feel, and become a hero instead of a victim in the story you tell."*
> — Fred Luskin

We all need to learn how to actively forgive others to continue along the road to self-enjoyment. Unfortunately, they don't teach forgiveness or restorative justice in school. Beyond the empty "I'm sorry" platitudes, we are socialized to never forgive and, especially, to never, ever forget. It's way more convenient to claim your identity as the "hurt one" so you never have to overcome your own baggage and evolve. That's why so many of us stay stuck in our dark story.

Romantic relationships are perhaps the most notorious playing fields for heartache, betrayal and unforgivable behaviour. Logically, we know that holding on to anger or resentment is like drinking poison and expecting the other person to be harmed. Even so, we can't help but feel justified for holding a lifelong grudge.

In my work with couples, I've learned it's entirely possible to let go of all the things that did not go as planned. If we find the learning or life lesson in relationship breakdown — the gift — this is often what leads us to a place of forgiveness.

My own experience of an ugly divorce with my first husband meant holding onto pain and anger for years. Anger and resentment are like quicksand — you get swallowed up in it. As for compassion, that's reserved for people who are deserving of it, right? At least that was my stance.

Now I look at that dark package and ask, "How did I ever navigate successfully through that trauma? Is there something I would do differently?" And with my second divorce I'm asking, "How can I continue to be on amicable, friendly terms with the father of my children?" I think that's a noble and worthwhile goal for all divorced couples with children. It's also important to consider, "How can I cultivate compassion for my ex-husband? How might that change the entire direction of my future and our children's futures?"

In March 2020, a few weeks prior to signing a legal separation agreement, I enrolled in family and marital therapist Katherine Woodward Thomas' course on "Conscious Uncoupling" — a program made popular by actress Gwyneth Paltrow's divorce proceedings.[23] I'd just read the chapter in Woodward's book on compassion, and I felt a warmth inside, a letting go — was my anger softening?

I had also stumbled upon a poem about compassion and forgiveness that had been adapted from a Christian prayer. Long Island divorce lawyer Wendy Samuelson recommended reciting this poem at the beginning of every divorce proceeding to demonstrate loving kindness for all parties. What a revelation! I learned how this practice had actually hastened the pace at which separation agreements had been signed and finalized.

Was I ready to forgive?

It seemed much easier to just hate your ex and wallow in self-pity than to accept responsibility for your role in the marital breakdown. I read the following poem over and over again to myself until I felt ready. Ready to have compassion for my ex-husband. Ready to forgive myself. Ready to finally move forward and negotiate a mutually satisfiable separation agreement.

MEDITATION FOR HEALING

Light before me
Light behind me
Light at my left
Light at my right
Light above me
Light beneath me
Light unto me

Light in the eyes of those who see me
Light in the ears of those who listen to me
Light in the hearts of those who think of me
Light in the hearts of those who speak of me

Light restore me to health
Light be always in my heart
Light be within me
Light establish me forever
Light be around me and preserve me
Light be before me and lead me
Light be within me and give me life
Light be near me and rule me
Light be beneath me and fortify me

I love the Light in those whom I may have
offended, knowingly or unknowingly
May the Light be with them
So be it
So it is
It is done

Adopted by Dr. Joseph Michael Levry from an ancient Christian prayer.

I now look at forgiveness as an effective way to release myself from anger and the desire to seek retribution.

Forgiving my ex-husband meant I could finally stop fantasizing about all the ways to make him suffer. I know it's hard to believe, but when you forgive others, you find freedom. I have also witnessed this transformation and positive outcome for hundreds of my clients and within my own friendship network.

So, as we round the corner toward Checkpoint 3 on this jam-packed road trip, I hope you will agree that we are all beautifully fallible. Learning how to grow beyond errors, to let go and forgive yourself, as well as others, is a vital step in achieving mental health resiliency.

Forgiveness is having the openness of heart to take a walk in another's shoes, while having the inner strength to take responsibility for your own role in the demise of any relationship. Compassion will always fuel forgiveness.

Of course, you have complete control over who, how and what you forgive. So, when you choose to forgive, you can also choose:

- Not to accept behaviour that has the potential to hurt you
- To leave a situation that is not healthy for you
- Not to have contact with those who have hurt you in the past
- Not to reconcile with the individual

The end goal is, of course, self-forgiveness and freedom. Breathe that in. All the buzzing of good endorphins — the releasing of those old, fractured stories — the full acceptance of your dark gifts.

Now, let's unpack and embrace everything that needs our focused attention and support at the next eight checkpoints as we move far beyond just surviving and learn the tools needed to be optimally thriving. Gas up, grab some more snacks and follow me.

PART THREE

EMBRACE
YOUR GIFTS IN DARK PACKAGES

CHECKPOINT 3

The Phoenix Fix

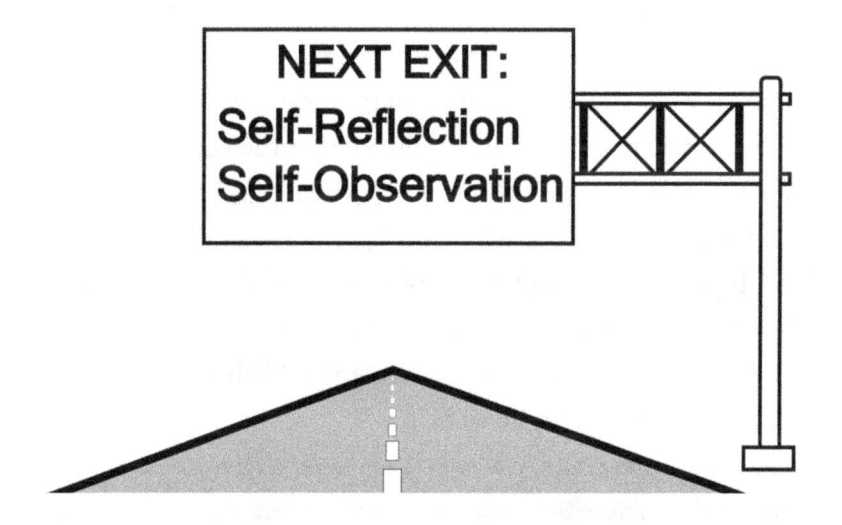

"It is during our darkest moments that we must focus to see the light."
— Aristotle Onassis

POWER OF SELF-REFLECTION

You've now made it through Checkpoints 1 and 2 on the Mental Health Resiliency Roadmap. Way to go! I hope you're learning and enjoying the ride home to YOU. There are lots of little practices to keep doing every day such as dipping into your mental health booster jar, repeating to yourself, "I'm here for you, everything will be okay and I'm never going to abandon you again," especially when dark packages show up. Also, practise self-compassion by only speaking to yourself in a kind, loving way.

So, the gas tank is full and we're back on the highway navigating Part Three together. It's time to completely embrace your dark gifts wherever you're at — right here, right now. I know it's hard to believe you could transform your life for the better. It can seem pretty impossible when you're feeling battered, bruised and lying in a pile of ashes. That's why Checkpoint 3 is called the "Phoenix Fix." If you give yourself permission to sit in the rubble and ashes of your life, that's where the magic happens.

Here's a client story about practising self-observation and self-reflection — at this highway exit.

Marissa had never been to see a counsellor before she arrived in my office. At sixty-two years of age and recently retired from a very successful career as an insurance broker, her life had taken a turn for the worst. Her husband of thirty-three years had announced he was moving to go live with his long-term mistress. Marissa's world came crashing down — burning ashes of what she had known to be her life were scattered all around her. She had dutifully moved with her husband across the country for his new job barely two years ago — just one of many destabilizing moves throughout their married life. Now, Marissa found herself with no husband, no job, no friendship network and no retirement hobbies. After years of attending to her husband's every need, she was now drowning in a sea of self-abandonment.

I listened attentively and validated Marissa's profound pain and concerns. Then I encouraged her to surrender to the firestorm that was now her life — feel the ashes at her feet — harness her fury. I suggested that, like the phoenix in Greek mythology, sometimes we have to fully embrace the flames that have engulfed our life — knowing that rebirth is the gift in that very dark package. So, that's what Marissa did — she channelled enormous energy from her anger and pain. It was an arduous therapeutic process, yet so worth it. Eventually, she found freedom of spirit in self-observation and self-reflection — a newfound joy that was all her own.

Little did I know, years later as a fifty-something woman, my life would also come crashing down in a self-abandonment firestorm. Like Marissa, I'm a high-functioning, high-achieving, serial codependent. What that means is I get into relationships with people I think I can fix, put the needs of others first and take care of their urgent life challenges as if they were my own. Being a therapist makes it even easier for me to intervene in stressful situations with incredible finesse.

Over the years, fixing others has been at the expense of my own physical and mental health – not to mention, my overall enjoyment of life. Do you recognize yourself here? My own pain and suffering kept getting pushed deep down inside — my joy put on hold. The thought was always, "I'll get back to me once I fix my partner's much more urgent problem. Then I'll rest, reflect and focus entirely on myself." Yet, I never stopped to ask myself, "Do I want a project or a partner?" So "me time" never came. Instead, I kept waking up in a relationship where I had lost all sense of self.

Three words — betrayed, bitter, angry — were stuck on repeat as the tidal wave of marital breakdown swallowed me whole. Anger filled my body, seething, rising like a raging inferno. I gritted my teeth and yelled, "Bring it on!" That's right, anger can be my best friend right now. Yes, anger is probably the most energetic emotion anyone can channel at such a time. I had helped so many women like Marissa to transform their lives. And now it was my turn to walk my own talk.

It was like I was being summoned to bear witness to my inner inferno of anger and ignite the rebirthing process — the Phoenix Fix.

And as we learned at Checkpoint 1, fully experiencing anger — an emotion that many of us try to dismiss, dress down, or disguise as sadness — is critical. In her book, *The Dance of Anger*, renowned psychologist, Harriet Lerner, reminds us, "Our anger often tells us that we are not addressing an important emotional issue in our lives, or that too much of our self — our beliefs, values, desires, or ambitions — is being compromised in a relationship."[24]

Guilty as charged. Unlike most men who are socialized to rise up, fight and openly express anger, women are revered for being docile peacemakers and are often condemned as "bitches" for expressing anger. I, like many of my female clients, was stuck in that "nice girl" loop where I'd accumulated an unconscious storehouse of anger and rage.

According to Lerner, we must experience anger, but not get stuck in the narrow story we tell ourselves about our mistakes. Otherwise, we stay in a continuous spiral — reliving the same story over and over again. We fan our own flames instead of rising from the ashes to embrace our dark gifts.

In Part One, we looked at this faulty conditioning — like believing that we can think our way out of experiencing adversity and destabilizing feelings. So, whenever we experience anger, instead of sitting with this emotion — observing and letting it inform us — we usually move to resolve this uncomfortable feeling as quickly as possible. How can we make it go away? Who can we blame? We rationalize our justifications for being angry then move toward a quick fix — an anger resolution.

Sound familiar? Unfortunately, this pattern doesn't prevent the next outburst, resolve the reason for the triggering experience or pave a way forward.

At this checkpoint, I want you to practise the Phoenix Fix by fully experiencing the weight and breadth of a stressful memory — feeling the emotional discomfort or pain — then taking time for self-reflection, readjusting your perspective and thanking this dark gift for its transformative power.

We will learn to say, "I no longer fear the darkness because I trust the phoenix in me will rise from the ashes and flourish."

Eventually, we will find ourselves at our rock bottom with no other choice than to embrace our darkness and dance within the flames. The Phoenix Fix is being fully present and allowing self-acceptance — which we practised at Checkpoint 2 — to inform you. It's saying, "Come on over here, anger. I've been waiting for you." Welcome these strong, powerful emotions by letting them surge throughout your body with fierce self-compassion.

Let's try Step One of the Phoenix Fix, now:

🎁 GIFT BOX RESILIENCY TOOLS

Acknowledge Anger/Forgive Yourself

1. Write in your journal or speak out, for at least three minutes without stopping, all of the ways in which the flames of a recent painful situation have affected you.

2. Take a deep breath and release the air through your mouth with a loud sigh.

3. Remember anger is an energetic, restorative emotion. Walk over to any mirror and tell the person in the reflection this: "I feel disrespected because _____ and I'm furious about _____."

4. Remember your forgiveness tools. Tell yourself, "I forgive you _____ (say your name out loud) for abandoning me. I love you unconditionally. I will help you honestly look at this situation and rise from the ashes and create a whole new ME. You got this _____ (say your name out loud)."

And that's the first big step in the Phoenix Fix because:

Pain + Reflection (new view of the situation) = TRANSFORMATION

This concept is the cornerstone philosophy of Ray Dalio, business investment guru, who teaches the importance of reflecting upon the pain of past failures in order to discover a whole new operating principle — a new maxim for life. The mistakes we make are the most transformative learning experiences — so much more than the sum of our successes!

Here's another client story to further demonstrate this concept:

Mary, an accomplished client in her late forties, is a good example of someone who realized a Phoenix Fix transformation. She was haunted by grief and self-directed anger after terminating a pregnancy in her early thirties. Although every woman should be able to decide whether to continue or terminate an unplanned pregnancy, it was a decision Mary ended up deeply regretting. She had difficulty with commitment in her intimate relationships, felt unworthy of love and couldn't let go of the thought that the abortion was the worst mistake of her life. By learning to finally acknowledge and experience these overwhelming negative emotions, Mary was able to start to create and believe a new story.

This new transformative story centered around an incredible woman who has helped countless children grow and prosper in her work with youth across the globe. Children she has birthed, loved and nurtured in a non-traditional parenting way. Children she continued to support and nurture just as any mother would do. Mary recognized the depth of her own feelings — empathy, sensitivity and self-love — that revealed themselves as the gifts in her dark package. There's no doubt she'd have been an amazing mother to her own biological child. But, she no longer doubted that she was a lovable person — worthy of intimate and loving connections with others. Mary realized the blessing in disguise was her legacy — the "extraordinary mother" she had become to hundreds of children who otherwise might not have had the opportunity to rise above their impoverished circumstances or overcome great adversity.

Simply put, the Phoenix Fix is a mindset-shifting tool.
The Phoenix Fix is deciding to feel all the emotions of your own "pity party" and then exit the room, knowing it's time to join forces with the "pivot party" crew. From experience, I can tell you the guests at the pivot party are way more fun — they have better snacks, belly laughs, party tricks and empathic listening skills. A pivot party doesn't mean you bypass the messy black hole of emotional work. You simply make the conscious choice to leave the pity party, reboot your mindset and turn your pain into something meaningful instead of wallowing in it forever.

Harold Kushner, a gifted rabbi, discusses this mindset shift in his book, *When Bad Things Happen to Good People*. Kushner describes the unimaginable pain of raising his son, Aaron, who was diagnosed with an incurable disease as a toddler. The disease caused Aaron to age prematurely and die at just fourteen years old. Kushner described this gift in a dark package — its emotional and physical pain — as the only reason why he became an extraordinary rabbi. His gift was the drive to reach millions of followers with a message of hope and renewal instead of merely living his life as what he calls a "mediocre" rabbi.[25]

What I want you to know is that you already have all the answers you'll ever need inside of you.

All you have to do is keep tapping into your emotions — the primary vehicle for informing those answers — your own personal Sherpa for life's ups and downs. Remember that you can choose to change how you feel at any time, so choose things that make you feel happier.

Step Two of the Phoenix Fix is simply deciding to feel a little bit better and have fun right now.
So, guess what? You can decide that you're deserving of joyful moments and happiness today. Right here, right now. You can choose one small thing this minute, this hour, this day that brings you a snippet of joy — like petting a dog, taking in the scent of an essential oil or staring at the sunset. I agree it can be really hard to flip that switch to feel deserving of happiness and joy. But the joy button is just sitting there waiting for you.

Yes, I know the drill — work first, play later. Who has time for joy? Many of us have been ruled by a strong work ethic that brainwashed us into thinking, "You must work very hard to survive, get your job done, finish literally everything and then and only then, can you play." We've been obsessed with outcomes — fixated on checking boxes — and achieving specific deliverables before enjoyment is ever granted. We don't let ourselves feel happy, satisfied or relaxed until we realize that outcome. If anything, we almost take pleasure in staying in the smoldering ashes of pain — in an absurd sort of way.

As I rework this checkpoint, I'm feeling unworthy and undeserving of the vacation I have booked on the Sunshine Coast of British Columbia with my two kids and my amazing friends. I'm finally returning after two years to the magical place that renewed my soul. Yet, I'm beating myself up for not meeting the unrealistic deadline I set for myself to have this book finished in less than six months' time. I feel like I should not be celebrating until my current project, this manuscript, is completed.

Let's officially detox from all of this self-sabotage and allow transformation to happen. How about scheduling in something fun today?

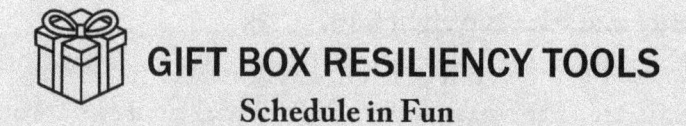

GIFT BOX RESILIENCY TOOLS
Schedule in Fun

1. Tell yourself to stop postponing your joy. You're ready to find and press the happiness button in your brain right now.
2. If you haven't already planned breaks in your day, please book out a fifteen minute break in both the morning and afternoon.
3. Make a list of any activities that make you smile or elevate your mood such as: singing or dancing to music, walking in the park, taking photos of flowers, playing with your pet, calling a friend who makes you laugh, decorating, etc.
4. Set a start time reminder notification on your phone and computer.
5. Before you start your "fun break" close your eyes and imagine sweeping away all the ashes that are keeping you stuck in "feeling bad." If need be, grab a broom and sweep the floor around you. I find cleaning always clears my energy.
6. Give yourself permission to feel good. Embrace the feelings of contentment and joy that will come from doing a little fun activity on your

> break. Say to yourself, "This is joy – bring it on!"
> 7. Enjoy yourself for ten minutes. Then quickly jot down or journal your mood shift.
> 8. Add more fun activities as you continue throughout the week and month, making this your new "Phoenix Fix Fun" activity — a non-negotiable moving forward in your life.

Of course, I appreciate that it takes courage, time and patience to incorporate something new in your life. It may not be easy to suddenly start adding in mood boosters if you feel overwhelmed. Feeling better often requires a range of coping tools and supports, especially if your whole life has been turned upside down or imploded. I get it.

Step Three: What to do if growing anxiety, panic and sleepless nights are stopping you from adopting a new mindset.
1. Book an appointment with your family doctor who may be able to prescribe a regimen to improve your sleep and mitigate your anxiety.
2. Complete a mental health assessment as suggested at Checkpoint 1.
3. Begin a self-reflection practice: journalling, meditation, gratitude. We will be exploring ways to do these practices at Checkpoint 5.
4. Reach out for support from a trained counsellor or psychotherapist.

One of the lesser-known counselling modalities that has helped me personally, rise from the ashes, is accelerated resolution therapy (ART). Developed in 2008 by licensed marriage and family therapist, Laney Rosenzweig, ART is a directive way to produce fast recovery from painful experiences in just a few sessions. It combines eye movement desensitization reprocessing (EMDR) and cognitive behavioural therapy (CBT) with guided imagery rescripting.[26]

With ART, the last of the burning ashes and stressful memories can be reprogrammed in your brain in a new, more adaptive way. It has been scientifically proven to literally rewire your brain — rework the memory of any traumatizing event — so it does not produce the same overwhelming visceral, emotional or physical responses anymore.[27]

So, it's kind of like being handed the remote control to create a more positive outcome in the feature film of your own life. For example, you can take a painful scene from your marriage, your childhood, or your workplace and rescript it with your own director's cut in one or two sessions. You're given creative licence to run people over or simply flood your brain with unicorns and daisies. Whatever works for you. It's cathartic neuroplasticity at its best.

My hope is that modalities like ART and other psychological treatments will become more readily available and accessible in the future. I encourage you to seek out and access whatever mental health supports work for you as we continue on the somewhat bumpy Mental Health Resiliency journey.

You can start by practising the Phoenix Fix tools today. They've been proven to help you safely manage the big bumps in the road and navigate detours along the way. So on those days when feelings overwhelm you, please know it's okay if you suddenly cry in Starbucks, or feel like throwing your cell phone against a brick wall. It happens. Don't forget to remind yourself that, "You are not your anger" – you're simply observing these outbursts from a safe distance and welcoming the learning and insight to come.

Doing the opposite — carefully orchestrated emotional control — will eventually unravel into burnout. Falling into the self-pity trap, which is frequently a delaying tactic to avoid taking responsibility, also stifles the opportunity for our greatest transformation.

The Phoenix Fix is knowing that we're only able to rise from the ashes and shine a new light on our situation because of the darkness.
— Catherine Clark

CHECKPOINT 4

Curb Your Catastrophizing

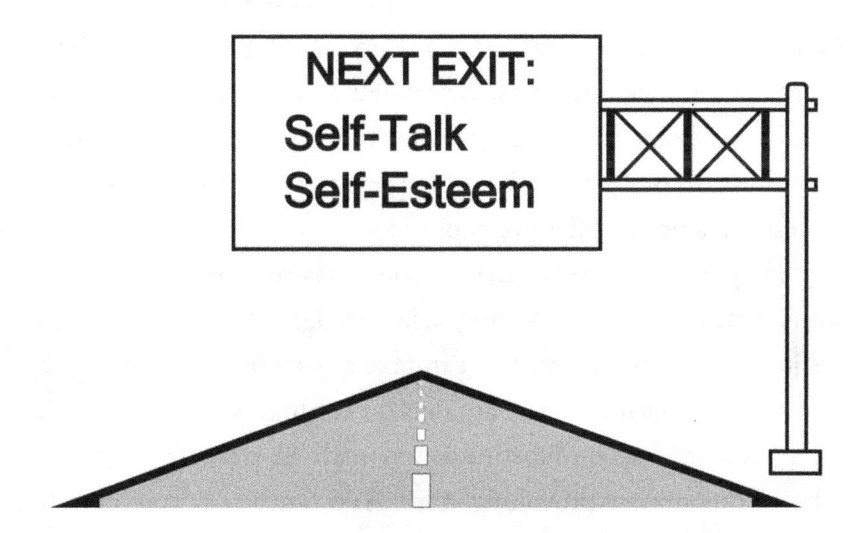

"Waking up is to expand our consciousness in all that we think, say, and do; liberating ourselves from old conditioning and all the mental constructs that underlie anxiety, tension and ego-driven demands."
– Deepak Chopra

As I approach the exit ramp, some idiot is riding my bumper. He's after me. I clutch the steering wheel, my hands wrapped so tightly around it that my nails dig into my palms. Breathing is hard — really hard. I speed up and the idiot does the same. OMG! That transport truck is going to run the light. I have no choice — I yank the steering wheel sharply to the right, mounting the curb and flying straight onto the sidewalk, panicked.

I blink my eyes and realize this incident never even happened.

This self-dialogue is an excerpt from a client's real-life experience of driving anxiety. It's a common occurrence. Usually, a person has experienced a car accident, or at least a close call, and that memory is still causing the subconscious mind to be protective. In other instances, anxiety can show up seemingly out of the blue — the appearance of crazy, overwhelming scenarios that only exist in our head. The more we try to stuff fear and dark memories deep down in our psyche the more they keep popping up because repression is not an effective coping tool.

The good news is you can curb your catastrophizing — whether you're driving or not — simply by acknowledging that your thoughts are just that — thoughts. You can take a deep breath, then say to yourself, "It's normal to feel anxious on the highway, but I know I can handle it." So, you substitute more realistic and affirming self-talk for the anxiety provoking story. And that's how you literally take back the wheel.

At this checkpoint, we will pick up the tools needed to reframe and craft more realistic self-talk — the messages you tell yourself about your stressors, past trauma and hardships. This self-talk is something we touched on at Checkpoints 1 and 2. Acknowledging your feelings and the story you keep telling yourself is vital to growing beyond your life challenges.

Change your story, change your life!

In fact, our mindset may be the most powerful tool we possess on the Mental Health Resiliency Roadmap. We become whatever we tell ourselves. For instance, we get whatever follows, "I'm a _____, bad driver, loser, success, good person, etc." Nothing forces us to reboot our mindset and let go of previous assumptions more than a full helping of adversity.

So, let's learn to recognize that our ego carries a story that can be rewritten over time. Neuropsychologists call these our schemata or core beliefs: a shortcut our brain has created like spyware. It's always operating unconsciously in the background. We just need to find the switch. That's right. We need to locate the automatic, adrenaline-pumping, survival mechanism switch and flip it to the off position. Then we can calmly talk back to our reptilian "fight or flight" brain saying, "Thanks for trying to keep me alive, but I've got this now," "I'm a good driver," and, "I know how to stay safe on the road."

Dr. Wayne Dyer, an American psychologist and motivational speaker, is well known for saying, "Change the way you look at things and the things you look at change."[28] Rooted in quantum physics, this concept is based on the fact that the way in which we actually observe particles, changes the particles. It follows, therefore, that the way we look at ourselves, observe a situation, feel our emotions (or not), or listen to our self-talk, will have a significant impact on how we experience life.

The glasses that we wear are also constantly being adjusted. For example, while I was working in the Arctic, I remember flying home to Toronto around Christmas time. I hadn't been in a car or on a highway for several months. As we approached the onramp to the 401 highway, it felt like my heart was beating out of my chest. My mind was spinning like a video game ready for combat.

I slouched in my seat to avoid watching the road. I was completely flooded. As a seasoned big-city driver, this response shocked me. My worldview had changed so drastically living in the wide-open tundra that the speed of city life became an assault to my senses. I had to immediately adjust my self-talk from a place of discomfort and fear to saying, "I'm safe, and I've driven hundreds of times on this highway without experiencing a serious incident."

So, we can reshape our perception at any time as difficult situations arise. We just need to switch on our affirming self-talk and remind ourselves of our survival stories.

In fact, anthropologists have long documented the importance of powerful storytelling as an antidote to catastrophizing behaviour. The consistent, cool headedness in everyday Inuit life is a good example of this behaviour. The Inuit view being angry or yelling at young children as unproductive. Instead, discipline is mostly taught through oral storytelling passed down from generation to generation. The Inuit have lived off the land for thousands of years. In order to survive, they had to regulate strong emotions like anger. They had to hunt, butcher the meat and make clothes from the skins — all of which takes an enormous amount of skill and attention. So, stories became the primary teaching aid for survival strategies and decatastrophizing tools.

At this exit, let's *stop* telling ourselves completely untrue stories that keep us stuck on autopilot — especially when the tape we play in our head is dictated by other people, places or things. Instead, let's *start* embracing our dark packages and all that we've survived up to this point.

The tools at this exit will help you do just that. I've witnessed the transformative power in action from these tools — even the tiniest micro-shift in perspective can shine a new light on your situation and move you from a place of powerlessness to self-control and self-confidence.

Let's learn about two of these mindset-rebooting practices now:
1. Locus of Control
2. Crooked Maladaptive Thinking

LOCUS OF CONTROL

> *"All that we are is the result of what we have thought."*
> — Buddha

Each of us exists on a continuum where we vacillate from an internal Locus of Control (LOC) to an external LOC as shown on the axis below. Can you identify where you might typically hang out on this axis?

External Locus of Control	*Internal Locus of Control*
<───────────────────────────	───────────────────────────>
Outcomes outside your control	*Outcomes within your control*
Determined by fate, independent of your own hard work or decisions	*The result of your hard work or decisions you have made*

Dr. Julian Rotter developed the LOC inventory in the 1950s to measure the degree to which individuals believe they have the ability to control what happens to them (internal) or how much they think that forces beyond their control affect their situation (external).[29] Rotter's concept has been used in marriage counselling, athlete performance maximization, stress management, employee hiring and leadership practices.

So, how can this concept help you? Knowing where you are on the LOC continuum will further uncover your spyware — your built-in self-fulfilling prophecy thinking — that affects your self-talk and overall self-esteem. For example, you either think you have the power to control whether you arrive on time for an appointment or you don't. Your expected outcomes continuously reinforce your future expectations and worldview.

In some societies, like Japan and China, people are encouraged to adopt more collective behavior, unlike in American society where individualism is more highly regarded. So, cultural LOC differences are certainly expected. Some people will possess both internal and external traits depending on their upbringing, the event and their circumstances. Then there are people who use external beliefs to justify failures even though they frequently exhibit an internal LOC. Go figure.

So, let's look at this concept a bit closer to see how we can apply it to our decatastrophizing behaviour. Can you identify yourself in either of the scenarios below?

External LOC
We all have that friend who is chronically late. Every time it happens, there's a litany of old excuses, such as the traffic was bad, my tire needed air, my alarm didn't go off, there was a fire in the metro, the coffee line-up was super long — the list goes on. If you think you might be late because you can't control your environment, this mindset gets reinforced over and over again and your lateness becomes even more entrenched. Are you that friend who blames external circumstances or everyone else for things happening in your own life? If yes, it's highly likely you're operating with an external LOC.

In my experience, a client with an external LOC will choose to let outside forces dictate their emotional state and self-worth. They're more likely to operate from a "victim" mentality, regularly joining their pity party friends in a chorus of blaming, criticizing, giving up and checking out. If they don't get a job that they're seeking, they'll often blame the company, unfair business practices, the economy or any other possible factor.

Sadly, someone with an external LOC also has difficulty taking credit for their own success. Even when they get that perfect job, they attribute it to luck. The good news is you can outgrow the pity party with greater self-awareness and positive self-talk.

Internal LOC

Then there's that friend who seems confident in her abilities, owns up, takes responsibility for everything she piled on you last week, but also takes credit for what she does well. This friend is operating with an internal locus of LOC — believing she's in control of her well-being and life outcomes. For example, someone with an internal LOC might say, "If I get this job, it's because I prepared for the interview, polished my resume and bolstered my social media presence."

You may also see yourself in the cohort of people who believe if only their circumstances would change, they'd be satisfied, happy and fulfilled. For example, if they got a new job, fell in love or had more money, then all of their problems would go away. Yeah, right.

You know as well as I do, that kind of thinking is a trap. It keeps us stuck in a loop of scarcity, negativity and powerlessness. It's one of the most common ways we give up our power — imagining we have no control or discounting all the positives about ourselves. Of course, we don't always have control over our circumstances (take the Covid-19 pandemic, for example), but we always have the power to change our perspective and how we look at any given situation from moment to moment. We still have a choice.

So, what am I saying here? With a little effort you can uncover your mindset blocks and practise adopting a more adaptive LOC. You can learn to feel more empowered — regardless of the adversity you are experiencing. All it takes are mini shifts in behaviour — such as leaving a half hour earlier — and mindset shifts like saying, "Everything is always working out for me," or, "I've got this."

Let's stop for a coffee and dig a little deeper into how to apply these principles.

COFFEE WITH CATHERINE

1. Decide where you fall on the Locus of Control scale. Be honest. More internal, external or mostly in the middle?
2. Do you have a different sense of control at home compared to at work? With your friends as opposed to your partner? What do you do so well that you implicitly trust yourself, your abilities and outcomes?
3. When your external environment blows up and sucks big time (e.g., you lose your job, car breaks down, boyfriend cheats on you, etc.) does your internal self agree, saying, "Yes, I suck!" Or can you see another way to look at the situation?

4. Are you able to move along the LOC scale to acknowledge life sucks right now, but you're still an amazing and capable person? In what situations are you able to say, "I've got this, I'm resilient, everything is 'figureoutable'?"
5. What disempowering words like "I can't" and "I'm trying/hoping" do you frequently use? The phrase I disliked the most growing up was "we'll see" that's simply a passive way of saying no. These phrases are the lies we tell ourselves and others.
6. Try replacing these disempowering words with empowering language like "I can," "I choose to," "I get to," "I'm willing to" or "I am capable of this." Say it with me now, "I get to write this exam" or "I get to pick up my kids" versus "I have to" language. Pay close attention to how empowering statements lay down new neural networks that gas up your self-esteem tank. It's like we just went through the car wash.

CROOKED MALADAPTIVE THINKING

> *"What a liberation to realize that the voice in my head is not who I am. Who am I, then? The one who sees that."*
> — Eckhart Tolle

The therapeutic and self-help work I enthusiastically support is firmly based in cognitive-behavioural and self-compassion theory. So, to curb your catastrophizing, you need to already have the tools from Checkpoint 1 (Self-Awareness, Self-Honesty) and Checkpoint 2 (Self-Acceptance, Self-Compassion, Self-Forgiveness) in your resiliency toolkit. Only then can you objectively look at the bottom of your dark box and say, "It's kinda dark, sad and lonely in here. Anybody have a flashlight?" The illuminated path to self-esteem and self-worth is only made clear when you're open and receptive to seeing it.

It's worth repeating that our negativity bias — our endless scanning of the environment for worst-case scenarios — is not our fault. But the problem is, we've developed faulty, unhealthy connections over time that signal the brain to release adrenaline to our system for things that aren't life-threatening. For example, an overdue report, shoes that don't match or a direct message (DM) that's been left on read. We easily can spiral into overreaction.

It's a sinking feeling that wallops your chest, pulling you down into a minefield of fear, spiralling out of control, heart racing, hands sweating, leaving you feeling light-headed and hyperventilating.

If you have ever experienced a panic attack or driving anxiety, this reaction probably sounds very familiar. People visit emergency rooms every day for what feels like a heart attack but is often a panic attack — a barrage of irrational, overwhelming thoughts that trigger our fight or flight response into overdrive. Remember, the body doesn't know the difference between a real or an imagined encounter with a bear.

Lifting the lid on our unconscious negative thinking has the capacity to bring us more relief than anything else — more important by far than accolades, possessions, accomplishments or relationships.

Reframing your automatic thoughts in a more affirming way is not a Jedi mind trick. It's intentionally choosing to engage in more adaptive, realistic self-talk. I often ask my clients to imagine a critic who sits on your shoulder — the voice of a bully, a hockey coach, a parent — and literally raise your hand and swat that critic off you. Doesn't that feel good?

Or better yet, you can use your self-observation tools from Checkpoint 3 to simply "observe yourself, observing the critic" in any given situation without reactivity or judgement. Listen for disempowering language from your critic. If you can't spot the automatic cognitive distortions, which have been ingrained since childhood, ask for help from a close friend or a trusted coach.

Here's a list of cognitive distortions you can mull over to pinpoint your critic's typical irrational thinking patterns: Which one is most familiar to you?

1. All-or-nothing thinking (statements that involve "always" or "never")
2. Discounting the positive while focusing only on the negative
3. Jumping to conclusions
4. "Should have" statements ("I shouldn't have said anything!")
5. Catastrophizing: viewing a situation or event as much worse than it is (drama queens, I see you)
6. Making something personal when it isn't (e.g., your manager forgets to invite you to a big meeting, but you insist it's because she dislikes you)

7. Emotional reasoning (decision-making based on feelings rather than facts)
8. Overgeneralizing
9. Labelling (e.g., you make a mistake on a report and call yourself an idiot)

Don't worry. We all have at least three or four of these distortions as our defaults. But once you start noticing all your irrational thoughts — trust me you've been repeating them forever — you can start substituting more affirming thoughts. With some guidance and practice, you'll be manifesting the things you want in life, rather than continuously reinforcing a negative narrative in your subconscious brain. You can overwrite old neural pathways containing low self-worth beliefs with realistic self-talk that turbo-boosts your self-esteem.

Believe it. There's so much good stuff to uncover in that dark package of yours. One of the books that I recommend regularly for thought substitution is David Burns' *Feeling Good: The New Mood Therapy*.[30] It has an easy-to-use thought chart that helps you track triggering thoughts, assess your feelings and observe your behaviour. With focused attention and maybe a little therapeutic support, your self-esteem tank will soon be overflowing again.

☕ COFFEE WITH CATHERINE

Okay, I need another vanilla latte. We're making really good progress here, but there's a big construction zone ahead. So, let's officially flick that critic off your shoulder and rewrite these negative self-talk statements together:

- I'm a failure — not true. I'm just frustrated and great changes in my life have come from failing.
- I'm powerless to improve my situation — not true. I have power and control over my choice to stay stuck or move forward.
- I'm worthless — not true. I'm being overly harsh and discounting all the positives. I've done lots of things that matter in my life. I matter.
- I don't get to be happy — not true. I create my own happiness and self-esteem.
- Nothing good ever happens in my life — not true. I'm just overgeneralizing, discounting the positives, etc.

Now ask yourself these questions to begin to reframe your current situation:

1. What's great about it?
2. What's funny about it?
3. What can I learn from this situation and do differently today?
4. How will this experience make a great story in years to come? (My all-time favourite.)

🎁 GIFT BOX RESILIENCY TOOLS

Here are some more actionable strategies to help you turn off your stubborn, automatic thoughts. I suggest that you monitor your irrational thinking over the course of a few days or weeks using the four-step *Rewire Compass Companion* outlined below (Worksheet downloadable at www.catherineclarkconnects.com).

This challenge helps you to look in all directions for evidence that refutes negative thought patterns, in order to rewire balanced self-talk. First, draw four columns in your journal:

- **Step 1: Look North.** For the next few days, record examples of negative self-talk or troublesome thoughts that come up. In the first column, write down the specific phrases that occupy your inner monologue.

- **Step 2: Look South.** Label each negative thought with the type of cognitive distortion that you are experiencing in the second column. Use the list provided on page 109.

- **Step 3: Look East.** Refute the distortion by generating one to three examples of situations or experiences that disprove this belief. Write down

> any facts or truths that logically demonstrate why the thought is a myth (untrue). Identify any external factors that may have contributed to the situation, including your upbringing.
>
> - **Step 4: Look West.** Act like a "wiser you" by playing the role of a compassionate friend who is in the exact same situation. What advice would you give? What would you say to encourage or comfort your friend? What's a more realistic thought?

BROADEN AND BUILD

Another helpful strategy is to observe how your stream of consciousness is often flooded with continuous negativity. Have you ever noticed that for every positive emotion you can think of in a situation there are at least three or four negative emotions? [31] Of course, that's because we're innately programmed to focus our attention on what's wrong with a situation. What I've noticed in my own life and in my practice with clients is that we can curb our catastrophizing by actively focusing on what's right and positive with any situation.

A theory proposed by Dr. Barbara Fredrickson in 1988 called "Broaden and Build" confirmed that we cope better if we focus our energy and really pay attention to things that are positive — what's working. In this way, we can reprogram our brain to not only take action with the negative, but also find positive meaning in any event — the gift. One of the questions that I regularly ask clients in therapy, is, "Are there any other ways to look at the situation — are there any positives that could come of this event?"

This mindset becomes a beautiful feedback loop where the more positive things you notice, the more you flourish, so the more you keep on attracting positive experiences. For example, if you meet a new friend on Zoom who interests you but makes you feel a little insecure, try finding three things that you like about this person or what they have to say. Fredrickson says the ideal formula for flourishing with positivity is three to one — three positives to one negative observation.[32]

TOXIC POSITIVITY

I want to make it clear that an adaptive mindset shift is also not about being positive all the time. It's okay to be negative. Sometimes we just need to sit in our pessimistic "Eeyore" world — wearing our old comfortable shoes and listening to the same playlist over and over again. I respect that.

In fact, there is such a thing as toxic positivity when people become obsessed with putting a positive spin on absolutely everything. Of course, there are pros and cons to every situation, including a pandemic. Yet, those who flood social media with only positive messages, can make it seem like you're not entitled to feelings of anger and frustration. And then there are social media influencers who make a business of promoting toxic positivity by posting only their best airbrushed photos, six-pack workouts and videos of their happy, exciting lives.

As discussed in Checkpoint 1, we all need to vent and express negative emotions like anger, sadness, anxiety and jealousy. Toxic positivity is ultimately a denial of reality, even if your thoughts are blowing things out of proportion. If you've been laid off indefinitely, that's a big life upheaval, regardless of whether you're still in good health or your husband has kept his job. I'd be freaking out, too! No amount of positive thinking exercises will change this truth.

Being told your thoughts and feelings aren't legitimate means you avoid embracing the darkness. Instead, you suppress all negativity, thereby exacerbating physical health problems and worsening your mental health.

People who demand positivity from others are simply unsupportive. Toxic positivity breeds the same kind of self-stigma we discussed at Checkpoint 1. This stigma can make people feel ashamed. It's like disallowing someone their viewpoint — completely negating their story. Brené Brown in her book, *Daring Greatly*, describes this self-stigma as "an intensely painful experience of believing that we are flawed and therefore unworthy of love and belonging — something we've experienced, done, or failed to do makes us unworthy of connection."[33]

That's just downright harmful, especially when you're already feeling overwhelmed and all alone. It's like calling your friend for empathy and instead you end up feeling judged and minimized. Toxic positivity is that family member who chastises you for expressing frustration instead of listening to why you're upset. Or my personal favourite dismissive platitudes: "We all make choices" or, "Can't you just look on the bright side of things?" An example of this behaviour would be telling a mother to just get over the death of her baby because she is fortunate to have other children. Toxic positivity can also be a form of gaslighting — a manipulation tactic used to make someone question their own reality and deny their thoughts, feelings and experiences. Toxic positivity is also a favourite tactic of bullies and abusive partners.

A big part of moving forward on the Mental Health Resiliency Roadmap involves wholeheartedly embracing this belief, "You are exactly where you need to be at this moment." So, even though you might feel like it's Groundhog Day — reliving the same spin cycle of thoughts over and over again — our body has actually never experienced the exact same moment twice. Every moment — including your darkest moments — offers opportunities to embrace new learning and a new way of thinking.

Let's take a deep affirming breath and give ourselves credit for all of the mindset shifts and resiliency tools we've tried so far. Remember, we can thrive without having to strive so hard.

In his book, *Metahuman: Unleashing Your Infinite Potential*, Deepak Chopra reminds us that every cell in our body already has the wisdom to tap into our infinite possibilities for us to evolve and get unstuck.[34] Let's face it — as human beings, we're constantly forced to adapt to our ever-changing environment (e.g., outside temperature, food supply, infectious diseases).

Traditional spiritual leaders tell us that if we can channel our inner awareness/knowing/intuition, we will naturally be able to get unstuck and tap into "life affirming" self-talk. One of the best ways to do this consciousness mining is, of course, a regular mindfulness and meditation practice. That's truly the secret to living a life with greater ease.

So, let's grab a few more snacks, fill up our water bottles and look at mindfulness practices at the next checkpoint.

"Pain is inevitable, but suffering is optional."
— Dalai Lama

CHECKPOINT 5

Surrender It All

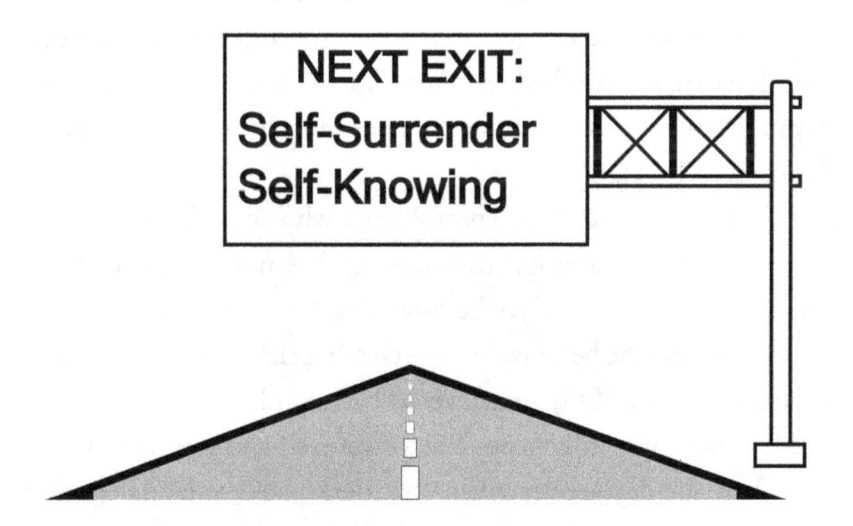

"When a train goes through a tunnel and it gets dark, you don't throw away the ticket and jump off. You sit still and trust the engineer."
— Corrie ten Boom

I used to be the kind of person who would hear the alarm clock and literally leap out of bed in the morning. I'd instantly check my phone and emails, watch the news updates, check the weather, check absolutely everything, unknowingly getting myself into a state of fight or flight — a frenzy of "do or die" adrenaline. I'd focus my attention on the struggle and the myriad of problems that needed to be solved that day.

What I now realize, is that how you start your day sets your intention, rhythm and basically the entire outcome of your day. When we wake up, reach for our phone and immediately disconnect from our bodies, it can cause a lot of dis-tress and dis-ease. So, what I do instead is call in thoughts of gratitude for another day on this earth, a warm bed and a restorative sleep. If you start your day in this way, you're guaranteed to feel more balanced and vibrant throughout the day.

As a caffeine-addicted control freak who embodies the phrase "hit the ground running," this strategy has not been a seamless transformation. And if you're anything like me, you've worked tirelessly to find the best practices — creating elaborately orchestrated strategies and skillfully maneuvered backup plans — to execute a comfortable, outwardly happy life for yourself and your family.

Then the day arrives when that dark package lands on your doorstep and you realize that all of the doing, thinking, planning and strategizing in the world is futile. You can't keep fighting. So, you finally give up on the illusion that you "should be able to" or "can" control everything. Even though we're conditioned to "never give up," you finally have to surrender — to stop fighting against or trying to change the here and now.

To be honest, that's not just a button you can push — sure wish it was. Although I've taken courses and even taught mindfulness workshops, it's still an up and down rollercoaster ride for me and most of the people I know. I'm still learning and practising right alongside you on this roadway.

All this "being" and "non-doing" business is tough slugging. I could barely get through two minutes when I first tried meditating because my mind was used to running an endless barrage of distractions like laundry, the grade five field trip form, a client PowerPoint, the grocery list, buying new snow tires, etc. But if this extroverted doer can live more mindfully, I guarantee you can too.

So, don't look at mindfulness as another goal to accomplish, but rather a mindset you invite into your life. And thankfully, when we have no other choice than to surrender — to sit still and trust — that dark package becomes the gift of self-knowing where you can flourish and thrive.

At this exit, let's clarify self-surrender and the role it plays in helping us embrace adversity. Let's shine a light on how mindfulness and self-knowing contribute to our mental health resiliency. Then we'll look at ways to cultivate mindfulness and pick up easy-to-use tools to integrate mindfulness meditation practices into our everyday lives.

Self-surrender and why we need it

Let's face it, sooner or later we all receive some news that brings us to our knees and rocks our very foundation. It may have been brewing for a long time such as terminal cancer or it may be a sudden event like a terrible car accident. Either way, we are pushed to our limit.

Surrender happens when you no longer believe or think you have all the answers. All you know is that you can't continue to operate as before. The game is up. You can't control the future or produce a guaranteed result. So, you give up, let go and release everything to a higher power beyond the egoic, thinking mind.

That's ultimately a good thing because self-surrender focuses your attention on the present moment like never before — the here and now. You relinquish control, which is necessary for living life with more ease, joy and less striving.

Self-surrender happens when you throw out your old GPS and trust this new boat on the river that will carry you wherever you need to go. Paradoxically, when you embrace this "not knowing" where life will lead, you tap into a higher self-knowing or deep well of insight — the dark gift. Although we can't just snap our fingers and decide to cultivate self-surrender and self-knowing, we can invite these traits into our lives. Mindfulness is one of the best vehicles to get us there. We can learn to "just be" — embrace life as it is now — to trust.

MINDFULNESS MEDITATION

"To the mind that is still, the whole universe surrenders."
— Lao Tzu

A common misconception is that mindfulness and meditation must involve chanting, sitting cross-legged for hours on end or embodying monk-like behaviours. I don't know about you, but after umpteen surgeries and body challenges, I can't do any of these things easily. In reality, mindfulness is a specific way of living that can be cultivated through practice. There's a category of meditative practices called "mindfulness meditation." These practices are a collection of disciplined exercises (some as simple as a morning gratitude, deep breathing, or guided visualization), that will help you cope with stress, manage your emotions, sleep better and improve your focus.

Jon Kabat-Zinn, renowned meditation expert and creator of the Mindfulness-Based Stress Reduction program (MBSR), describes mindfulness as, "Paying attention on purpose, moment-to-moment, without judgement."[35] When a deluge of thoughts pop up, as they naturally will, you simply acknowledge this as normal and shepherd those thoughts back down the mountain, as you continue to climb into "presence."

The bottom line is that mindfulness is the simple act of paying attention and being present in whatever you do. It fosters self-surrender and self-knowing — skills that you otherwise only achieve the hard way, with a full-blown breakdown. A meditation practice is just one of the many roads to mindful living.

Tim Ferriss, author of *The 4-Hour Workweek*, noted that an estimated eighty percent of the world's most successful people have a daily mindfulness practice.[36] These practices ranged from timed meditations and yoga to using an app like Headspace or Insight Timer (a personal favourite of mine).

Of course, adopting some of the daily transcendental meditation practices of monks, which Jay Shetty discusses in his book, *Think Like a Monk,* doesn't hurt either. Monks have been shown to have some of the highest gamma brain waves in the world, which are correlated with greater focus, memory, learning, inner peace and overall happiness.[37] Who doesn't want more of that?

As meditation expert Craig Krishna explains, "Meditation builds neuroplasticity — loosening those old nerve cells — to make space for the new ones to emerge. Meditation, in this sense, is a fire that burns away the old, conditioned self, known as the *Yajna* in the *Bhagavad Gita*."[38] Canadian psychologist Donald Hebb, who coined the phrase, "Neurons that fire together, wire together," also found that the more we practise mindfulness, the more we develop neural pathways in the brain associated with being "fully present."[39]

To me, mindfulness meditation is all about your inner world — embracing your dark shadows — and tuning into your "inner knowing" instead of all that brain chatter. It's getting rid of that incessant critic nattering in your mind once and for all.

Mindfulness is noticing the difference between "thinking-focused" behaviour — repeating the same words, feelings, opinions, justifications and phrases over and over again — and connecting to our calm centre within. It's being so actively, attentively focused on the present moment that thoughts of the past and worries of the future simply melt away. Of course, this has always been a part of the ancient lessons of Buddhism, as well as other eastern and indigenous religions.

Mindfulness has experienced a resurgence recently because many renowned spiritual teachers are freely sharing their knowledge online. Teachers such as Deepak Chopra, Eckhart Tolle, Pema Chödrön and Sarah Blondin guide us in surrendering to suffering and truly opening our hearts to experience joy. And we all need an extra helping of joy!

Eckhart Tolle, author of *The Power of Now*, is considered the "contemporary guru" of this spiritual awakening. He views suffering as a form of anger, depression, isolation and desolation. When you're stuck, he notes the primary cause of unhappiness is never the situation, but your thoughts about it — how your egoic mind views the situation.[40] So, meditation can help you become acutely aware of your thoughts — to see the thinking mind as separate from the situation, which is always neutral. It also reinforces the automatic thought-stopping techniques that we practised at Checkpoint 4.

If we can fully surrender to what's inside our dark package — get painstakingly immersed — completely still — we will be propelled toward greater self-knowing.

For me, mindful meditation is like a giant yellow mood-reset button. You can push it anytime that you need to clean your slate — breathe — and be fully in the now. Honestly, if you're a foodie like me, just stopping to engage all your senses in a freshly baked, warm scone topped with freshly picked, bright red raspberries and a dollop of crème fraîche is practising mindfulness. Just pause for a moment and sit with that yummy thought. Mmm.

How can we be more present and mindful?
Eckhart Tolle recommends practising being as intensely conscious of the "now" as we are in any emergency. For example, when I arrive onsite for a trauma intervention, I naturally let go of ego and fear to become acutely present and ready for whatever arises moment-to-moment in the situation. Then my best, most authentic self becomes laser-focused on being fully with someone who is in shock. Because it's only when we are engaged in the "now"— entirely present — that we can allow an otherwise unbearable incident to wash over and inform us.

Another way to become naturally engaged in the "now" occurs when we're walking in nature.

There's a magical forest trail on the Niagara Escarpment that I used to walk when I was moving through the darkness of depression. I remember that particular spring in vivid detail. New life was bursting forth everywhere. I credit my re-emergence and healing to the forest magic and my immersive, meditative walks. This moment was my first conscious experience with the mindfulness of nature and its resiliency lessons.

The forest teaches us that death is nourishment; that there is light in the shadows, renewal will find its season and joy is omnipresent.

The first time that you go on a mindful nature walk, you are overcome by awe and appreciation of the view. Later, as you fully immerse yourself in each walking moment, you notice all the tiny details of the landscape — skipping over a knotty root, becoming connected with a wise hundred-year-old tree, being intrigued by the subtleties of a cardinal, listening to the wind stir through the river — it's a mindful awakening. Returning again and again, you notice more and more: the ripple-like shadows that hover beyond the shapes of the trees, the dancing light in the stream, the intricate points on a leaf and the patience of the silent rolling hills.

When you lose yourself in the process of being, creating and feeling totally in "flow," you're experiencing mindfulness.

Many of my friends are highly creative beings who have told me that they have no need for a formal meditation practice. When doing their art — painting, gardening, singing, playing the piano, writing — they're fully present and lose all track of time in their craft. Working with your hands — in a state of creative bliss — is indeed a form of mindfulness and self-surrender. Even washing the dishes, folding clothes, knitting, practising your golf swing, refinishing a piece of furniture or riding your bike through the neighbourhood are forms of mindfulness.

You see, it's not so hard! Many of you already practise mindfulness without even knowing it.

Establishing a disciplined mindfulness practice in 2020 probably saved my mental health when Covid-19 brought our lives to a halt. The world was suddenly a very scary, unpredictable place. The only constant in my life was waking and completing my mindfulness morning practice — experiencing the freedom and power to create a new life for myself. Instead of obstacles and frustration, I saw possibilities and new opportunities. This practice is how I truly learned to embrace self-surrender more fully.

I could acknowledge the only thing keeping me in the dark, was myself — my egoic mind. If my mind started ruminating in the past or making noise about the future, I would read or listen to a passage from *The Power of Now*. To quote Eckhart Tolle, "Always say 'yes' to the present moment. What could be more futile, more insane, than to create inner resistance to what already is? What could be more insane than to oppose life itself, which is now and always now? Surrender to what is. Say 'yes' to life — and see how life suddenly starts working for you rather than against you."[39]

Over the past couple of years, I've expanded my awareness and self-knowing. I've become a full participant in my life again, tapping into love, joy and creativity that I had bypassed for years. Everything feels possible again. The final piece of the mindfulness puzzle for me was to set clear intentions— with honesty and clarity — for my deepest desires. While still living in Calgary, Alberta, I made a vision board with a photo of the Toronto CN Tower and a picture of the book that I was planning to write in 2021. *Et voilà!* Here I am, looking at the amazing view of the CN Tower and Toronto skyline from my top floor balcony while holding a foam core mock-up of my book cover.

When you shed your limiting beliefs and become fully present in your life, you can literally manifest anything.

Starting a Mindfulness Practice

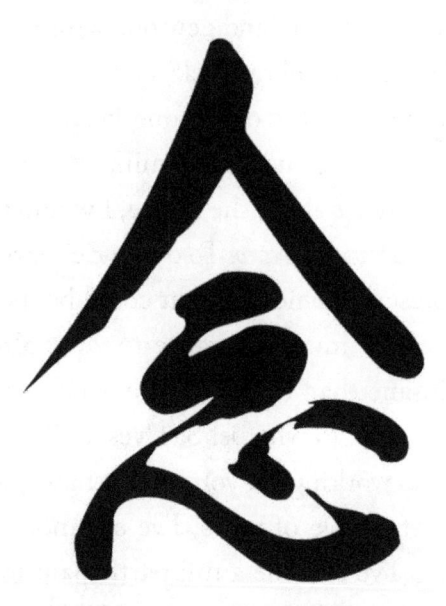

The Japanese character for mindfulness literally translates as "present heart." It is the practice of paying careful attention to what is happening in the now, whether it be a sight, sound, taste, smell, sensation in the body, thought or emotion. It is observation without attachment or judgement. The top strokes are suggestive of a roof or shelter and symbolize the "now" of the present moment. The strokes below the "roof" elements represent the heart or mind. Taken as a whole, this symbol can be interpreted to mean "being full-hearted (mindful) right now."

Here are three easy techniques that I suggest you adopt to have a "present heart," add to or build your mindfulness practice, namely, breathwork, gratitude and journalling.

Breathwork

We can mindfully escalate and de-escalate by harnessing the power of our breath:

- Learning how to take slow, deep breaths into your abdomen each morning is a delicious way to start your day or calm your body at any time.
- Breathing through your nostrils, concentrating on the air temperature as it enters cool and exits warm, is a great way to start mindful breathwork.
- Counting to four while breathing in, then making your exhalation twice as long by slowly blowing air out through your mouth, as if you were blowing through a straw, is a great way to engage the autonomic nervous system.
- Slowing down and deepening our breath lowers our heart rate to calm our body and mind. Deep diaphragmatic breathing helps settle the nervous system and calm the vagus nerve that is responsible for the regulation of internal organ functions, such as digestion, heart rate and respiratory rate, as well as vasomotor activity and certain reflex actions.

🎁 GIFT BOX RESILIENCY TOOLS

Anytime you feel overwhelmed, ask yourself this question: Is your mind full? Are you able to be mindful instead?

- Firstly, notice and follow your breath as we just discussed.
- I'm going to walk you through a 5-4-3-2-1 technique that I use to help ground clients who are having an anxiety attack (see the following downloadable chart).
- Purposefully take your mind off any uncomfortable thoughts and focus instead on the details of your surroundings. Use each one of your senses with intention, allow yourself to stop, be and experience the here and now.
- Please get up from your desk or where you are right now and step outside if possible — even stand in a doorway or on your balcony.
- Take a deep breath in on the count of four then slowly release it through your mouth for a count of eight. Repeat. Focus on the present moment with all five of your senses starting with five things you can see.
- Use the 5-4-3-2-1 technique below to ground yourself in the present moment. Name what you see, feel, hear, smell and taste to feel grounded and calm in the present.

Stay grounded using your 5 senses

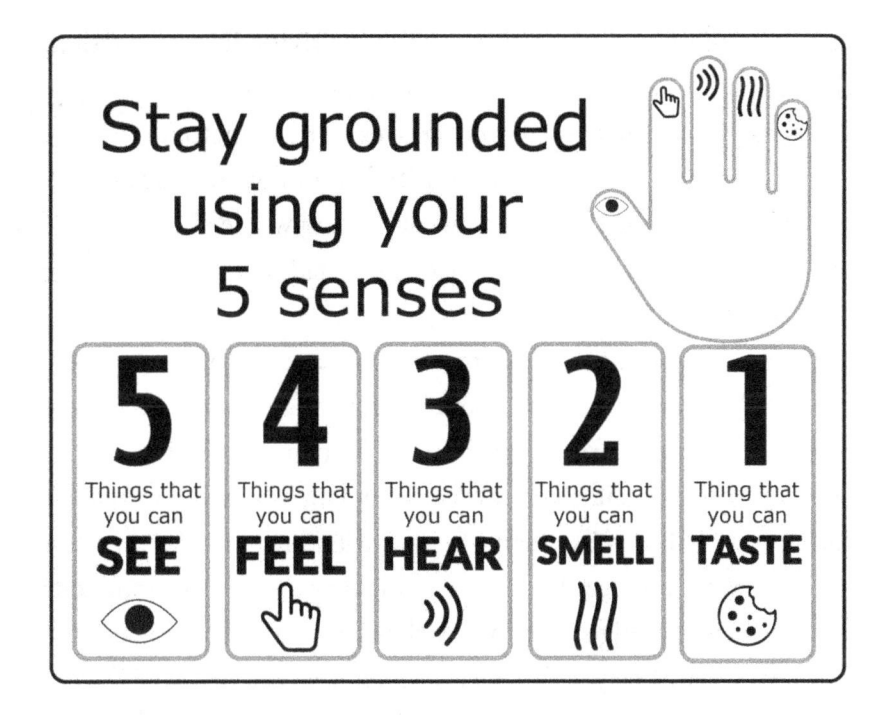

- **5** Things that you can SEE
- **4** Things that you can FEEL
- **3** Things that you can HEAR
- **2** Things that you can SMELL
- **1** Thing that you can TASTE

Gratitude

*"Wear gratitude like a cloak,
and it will feed every corner of your life."*
— Rumi

Gratitude is a mental health goldmine. Practising daily gratitude can help you shift your focus from complaining about hardships and what you don't have to acknowledging what you do have. Research has shown that one positive thankful interaction every morning has the power to set your entire day on a more positive path.

Gratitude has been linked to better mental health, self-awareness, better relationships and an overall enhanced sense of fulfillment. It also helps us to feel less resentment and pain. Several scientific journals, including the *Harvard Business Review*, have also reported that gratitude increases positivity, job satisfaction, risk-taking for innovation and, of course, resilience. Quite simply, it makes our personal and working lives so much better.

As a mindfulness exercise, gratitude grounds you right smack in the middle of the "now" — you can't be anywhere else — even if you try. It can instantly take you from your sad pity party to feeling thankful for all of your pivot party friends.

Mindfully saying thank you is the most basic way to acknowledge your gratitude. When saying thank you for a thoughtful, hand-made birthday gift from a friend, go the extra mile to describe everything you love and appreciate about the gift in detail. Sending a detailed thank you card or voice memo to your friend means that they can more fully experience the time, kindness and effort put into your gift. This acknowledgement enables the giver to feel fully appreciated and loved. Jay Shetty calls this the "feedback loop of love."[37]

You can show your gratitude with small acts of kindness — buying someone a coffee, volunteering, helping a friend — that helps entire communities to be more resilient.

GIFT BOX RESILIENCY TOOLS

Tips for Practising Gratitude

1. For one week, take a few moments at the end of each day to reflect, acknowledge and write down three things you are grateful for and why. Some families practise gratitude as they sit down for a meal at the kitchen table. Others see gratitude as a form of prayer, pausing to give thanks that there is food on the table or for good health.

2. Consider all the people with whom you interacted today. Recall what happened when you took a few moments to thank those on your path: the call centre employee, Amazon delivery person, coffee shop barista or executive assistant who fixed your PowerPoint?

3. Instead of focusing your attention on what you've lost, be grateful for what you have left. You have a choice to live every moment in gratitude as a gift.

4. Keep a gratitude journal. The week before you start this exercise, write down how much sleep you were able to get each night, then compare this number with your restorative sleep after you have completed one week of gratitude journalling.

Journalling

> *"Appreciate everything, even the ordinary.*
> *Especially the ordinary."*
> — Pema Chödrön

Journalling is a proven mindfulness practice that aids you in processing and reflecting on the day's events. By cataloguing the positives in your world, it can help you to reframe stress and adversity, not as pain, but as a challenge that you can process and deal with as it comes. Journalling for just five minutes a day encourages you to clear out unwanted thoughts — like a toothbrush for the mind.

The physical act of writing activates the analytical and rational left brain. As a result, the left brain is focused and busy, freeing the right brain to create new options or ways to see the day's events. Many executives that I've worked with have realized great success by starting each day with intention-setting — writing in their agenda three goals they intend to accomplish that day and creatively brainstorming the steps and supports needed to make this happen.

Future-self journalling is another type of intention-setting practice that helps you break out of your subconscious, conditioned mind and manifest a joyful, affirming future.

GIFT BOX RESILIENCY TOOLS

Future-self Journalling

1. Visualize yourself achieving an important goal/wish in the future. Write down the goal you desire (e.g., bestseller list, amazing life partner, financial prosperity) in specific detail by saying, "I am grateful for _____" as if it already happened.

2. Write down all the feelings and emotions (pride, joy, excitement, peacefulness) that come from having accomplished this goal as if it were really happening right now. Smile, breathe, take it all in, and feel the emotions with your whole mind, body and spirit.

3. Pause and think about what, if anything, might be in your way. Identify any obstacles inside that might prevent you from accomplishing this goal in the future (fear of success, imposter syndrome, lack of funds). Write these obstacles down.

4. Set a conscious daily intention to tackle each obstacle and then visualize one small and specific step you can take to move toward your future vision. (e.g., get up one hour earlier every day to write 500 words for my book).

> 5. Surrender your attachment to this goal or deep desire as though you've placed an order online to the universe and cleared all the obstacles for a successful delivery. Keep focusing on the little things that bring you authentic joy and peacefulness in the now.

MORNING ROUTINE (RINGS)

> *"The secret of health for both mind and body is not to mourn for the past, worry about the future, or anticipate troubles, but to live in the present moment wisely and earnestly."*
> — Buddha

My Current Best Practices
When we pulled over at this exit, I told you how the first ten minutes of your day sets the tone for how the rest of the day unfolds. So, the worst thing that you can do is to pick-up your cell phone and start aimlessly scrolling.

I start each day with a mindful morning routine so that I can visualize and put in motion inner calm, empowerment and a positive mindset. I start my day by saying an affirmation, setting a positive intention, doing breathwork and writing down three things that I'm grateful for in a dedicated journal. I then drink a large glass of water and take fifteen minutes to meditate, either a guided meditation or simply sitting in silence. Next, I stretch and scan my body for any parts that need some extra self-care. Weather permitting, this practice is followed by a twenty-minute power walk listening to my favourite podcast or audiobook.

Mindfully eating breakfast and drinking a fabulous cup of coffee are also integral parts of my morning routine. The first hour of my day is dedicated to sacred "me time." But even squeezing in just ten minutes for yourself to start a mindfulness practice is a positive step forward.

My morning routine is the one commitment that I've been able to keep for over a year. It's purposely setting out to support mental health resiliency from the moment your alarm rings. Not checking your cell phone for messages means you're not being immediately pulled into other people's agendas with all that reactivity and stress. You can respond to the needs of others once you've turned your "work mode" switch to the on position. Of course, many of us have partners, children and families to support during our mornings. That means you must start your day earlier, before the rest of your household is awake. Rising earlier makes you feel like you have so much more time in your day.

I suggest that you consider starting your day with quiet contemplation to support a balanced, calm mindset. I challenge you to take an honest account of what your current morning routine looks like and whether you're setting yourself up for a day with ease — or a day with dis-ease. It's important to also create a dedicated, sacred space in your home where you can consistently go to practise mindfulness. Personalize this space with the things you find pleasing such as a cozy meditation cushion, blanket, soft lighting, diffuser or candles to set the mood, journalling, unwinding and recharging your batteries.

And while we're at it, let's take a look at your nighttime routine as well. This routine is called "sleep hygiene" — another necessary mindfulness ingredient in your mental health resiliency toolkit. It's super important to find ways to unwind and draw a line to signify the end of your workday. Rituals like a bath or cup of tea, meditation music and shutting off all electronic blue light devices, can have a hugely positive impact on your ability to fall asleep and stay asleep. Did you know that your brain needs at least an hour to decompress and slow the neural network activity spike caused by using our devices? So, if you want to sleep at 11:00 p.m., I'd suggest that you turn off all your devices by 10:00 p.m.

If you're just considering a mindfulness morning routine for the first time, I highly recommend an app like Insight Timer, Calm or Headspace, or watching a YouTube video to get you started with even five minutes in the morning or evening. You may also visit my website for a free Magnetic Morning Meditation, Abundance Affirmations or Loving Kindness Meditation.

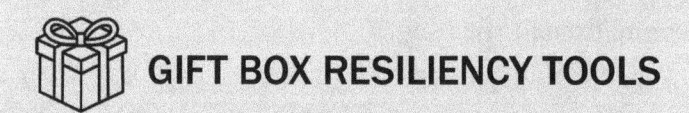

GIFT BOX RESILIENCY TOOLS

My Mindful Morning Routine

When the alarm rings, instead of leaping out of bed, try this RINGS acronym instead. You can lie in bed, move to a yoga mat or sit on a chair for this short mindfulness practice. Close your eyes, breathe and wrap yourself in a warm kaleidoscope of sight, sound and touch as you experience self-surrender and listen for self-knowing.

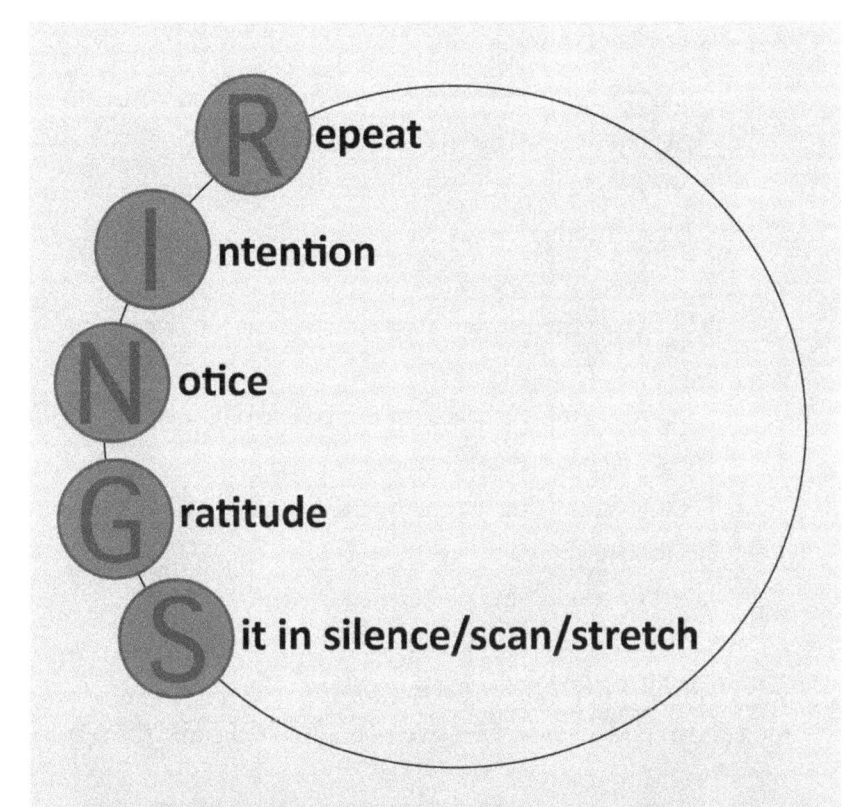

R — epeat
I — ntention
N — otice
G — ratitude
S — it in silence/scan/stretch

R — REPEAT an affirmation or mantra upon waking:
- "Everything is always working out for me."
- "Good things are coming to me today."
- "I am enough."
- "I am resilient."
- "I ROCK!"

I — INTENTION set for the day:
- How do you want your day to feel and unfold? Place your hands on your heart and imagine sending love, light and energy for that intention everywhere you may venture today.

- Visualize one to three important goals you will have completed by the end of the day.
- These goals are promises you're making to yourself today — say, "I've got this!"

N — NOTICE the present moment by fully engaging in the now:
- Follow your breath as it comes in and out of your nose. Repeat several times.
- Name one thing you can see, feel, hear, smell and taste.
- Feel grounded in the here and now.

G — GRATITUDE for having another day on this earth, for a warm bed and a restorative sleep. Journal three things every morning:
- Write down: "I am grateful for the opportunity to learn a new way to calm my body, mind and spirit each morning."
- Select one person for whom you feel deeply grateful today — write down why.
- Visualize a small kindness or helping hand someone is offering you today and write about the gratitude you feel.

S — SIT IN SILENCE, SCAN and STRETCH
- Go to the same spot every day to sit on a meditation cushion, yoga mat or chair.

- Sit in silence, select a guided meditation of your choice or set a timer (with a soft gong/chime) and dedicate as little as five minutes to closing your eyes and simply focusing on your breath. Acknowledge your thoughts and gently release them as you bring your attention back to your breath — the present moment.
- Scan your body for any pain or places where you may be holding yesterday's emotions. Send love to your beautiful body by thanking it for carrying you throughout your life.
- Stretch and hold the parts of you that are tight. Choose your favourite yoga poses as you spread positive healing energy throughout your body.

COFFEE WITH CATHERINE

Let's enjoy a morning coffee together before we get back on the road and head to Checkpoint 6, where we will ensure you get the self-care that you need to keep moving along the roadway toward self-fulfillment.

1. I'd like to talk with you about your dark gifts. Tell me something that you were not at all grateful for when it happened (job loss, relationship breakdown, health issue, work stressor, etc.).

2. Now I'd like to know the dark gift in this adversity — what did it teach you about yourself that you didn't know before? What have you learned that you otherwise would never have known about yourself?

3. What role did self-surrender or mindfulness play? Have you had a spiritual transformation — post-traumatic growth? Did you develop a deeper relationship or a new skill or strength as a result?

4. In what way is this experience worthy of your gratitude now? Let's take a moment to name it. "I'm thankful for _____."

"Enlightenment is always there. Small enlightenment will bring great enlightenment. If you breathe in and are aware that you are alive — that you can touch the miracle of being alive — then that is a kind of enlightenment."
— Thich Nhat Hanh

CHECKPOINT 6

Off-Balance

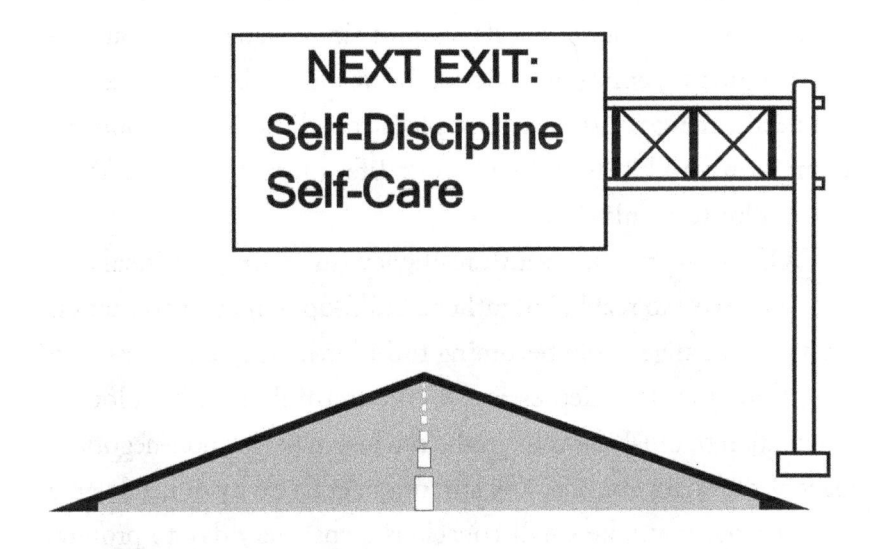

"Most of us spend too much time on what is urgent and not enough time on what is important. You have to decide what your highest priorities are and have the courage — pleasantly, smilingly, unapologetically, to say 'no' to other things. And the way you do that is by having a bigger 'yes' burning inside."
— Stephen R. Covey

LOVING USE OF TIME

Oprah Winfrey opens each of her famed *Super Soul* podcasts by saying, "The most valuable gift you can give yourself is the gift of time — time to nurture the unique spirit that is you."

The dark gift of the Covid-19 pandemic was that it forced people worldwide to take stock of what truly matters — what nurtures and sustains overall well-being. It gave us the dark gift of lockdown. It also shone a light on how we spend our valuable time — the balancing act needed for good mental health. This recalibration requires continuous self-discipline, self-care and checking in every day to see if you have air in each one of your four tires: cognitive, emotional, physical and spiritual. And, of course, we need caring relationships: a place to call home, a supportive community and a disciplined work/life integration plan. Wow, that's a lot to think about.

Of course, mental health resiliency isn't a singular ideal state that you strive to reach, but rather a build-up of many little actions that prevent anger from becoming full-blown rage, or sadness from spiralling into deep depression. Come to think of it, it's a lot like meditation or brushing your teeth. You just make it a non-negotiable part of your daily routine. You still might get a cavity or need dental surgery, but you take small conscious steps every day to promote oral health and prevent disease.

For many of us, the blurring of work-life boundaries is a growing mental health concern. More and more jobs have moved from office towers to "home offices." Home boundaries have become physically blurred. Bedrooms have become offices and study spaces, while still a place to rest our head and sleep — further blurring work-rest boundaries.

The growing burnout rate — another dark gift — has made us question our mobile office 24/7 availability mindset. Recent studies have found that North Americans are now working harder and longer hours — in many cases two-and-a-half hours more per day than before Covid-19 with wireless devices and Zoom. Even if you haven't been mandated to work from home, there is a growing realization that time is, indeed, our most precious commodity.

Happy, resilient people know it's your discerning use of time that makes all the difference. It's also what helps you bounce back quicker from any adversity. I often hear workshop participants and clients remark, "If only I had more time during the day, I'd get so much more of what matters to me done and I'd be so much happier." But would you really?

Stephen Covey, in his book *The 7 Habits of Highly Effective People*, makes the case that you must get crystal clear on your "Big Rocks" — the things that are super important to you — your non-negotiables.[41] We have many rocks, both big and small, which we must prioritize each and every day if we're to fit everything in our work-life integration jar. Most things can fit in the jar — the urgent, the unimportant and even the low priority. But the big rocks will only fit in the jar if you tend to them first. For example, you have to have the self-discipline to meditate and exercise first thing in the morning. Because before you know it, your day is jam packed with competing demands, leaving no time for your true priorities — relationships, professional development, exercise, eating healthy and sleep.

Dr. Robert Brooks, a Harvard medical expert in resiliency research, calls self-discipline one of the most vital components of a resilient mindset. We all know self-discipline means staying focused on your goal, problem-solving better and remaining in control of your reactions. But did you know self-discipline also means being good at saying no and delegating tasks?

Of course, it takes lots of practice to flex your "no muscle" until it becomes second nature. And for most of us, that's uncomfortable. But it's the best way to tackle the time vampires that can keep you stuck in an unhealthy, dark place.

Of all the bank campaigns that I worked on throughout my first career as an advertising executive, the single most memorable tagline was, "You're richer than you think." This message stood the test of time — through recessions and personal debt crises — and aired for several years. The campaign's emphasis was on carefully managing and maximizing the money that you have — an abundance mindset — and being self-disciplined, rather than adopting a scarcity, "never enough," mindset that keeps you in low productivity mode and financial self-sabotage.

To that end, imagine you have a "time" bank account that credits you with 86,400 seconds of time every morning. Twenty-four hours later whatever is not used for good purpose is lost. This "time" bank account does not carry a balance or offer overdrafts or cash advances. Each day, a new account is opened, and each night, the old account is closed. Your loss is your failure to use your twenty-four-hour allotment as lovingly and wisely as possible. Would you manage your time and focused attention any differently? I'm not so sure.

At this exit, let's consider how precious our daily fund of hours, minutes and seconds is to our overall health, self-enjoyment and self-fulfillment. Let's not wait until we're completely burnt out and falling up the stairs of some old hotel. Now is the time to take stock. I've squandered and given my time away needlessly for many, many years. That's why I'm grateful for my breakdown — the gift of time — and the insight I gleaned to write this book and relaunch my life.

I'd like to show you how to do the same. So, as Oprah recommends, let's unwrap the gift of time and pick up new strategies for self-discipline and self-care practices. Oh, and let's build in extra time for our coffee chats and maybe even a wine and cheese date.

WORK-LIFE INTEGRATION

> *"We need to do a better job of putting ourselves higher on our own 'to do' list."*
> — Michelle Obama, former First Lady

Amen to a former First Lady for reminding us to put our own name on the top of our "to do" list. At this highway exit, we'll need to clearly delineate work time from our leisure time and carve out time for self-care if we want to continue on this mental health resiliency mission.

Right now, the lines between focused work time, downtime, play time, sleep time and other ways that we spend our time have become very fuzzy for many of us. Yet, there's hope. I'd like to help you draw your line in the sand with fierce self-compassion. I have a multi-tool screwdriver to add to your "self-discipline" kit that just might do the trick.

Let's face it, the concept of work-life balance is good in theory, but it just becomes one more thing on our "to do" list — another unrealistic goal. There are two reasons why it seems unattainable: firstly, a lack of time and scheduling conflicts, and secondly, we feel overwhelmed, overloaded and stressed by the pressures of multiple roles. If you're part of the "sandwich generation," you're probably struggling to juggle your career, childcare and home-management on top of caring for aging parents. All it takes is one more dark package — like a child with a life-threatening illness or a parent with Alzheimer's — to stop you in your tracks and make you realize that you aren't invincible. Yikes! Let's bid an official goodbye to Wonder Woman.

One of the most requested corporate wellness workshops that I facilitate teaches resiliency, more specifically, work-life balance. The latest term is "work-life integration" because, as we know, even the concept of "balance" stresses people. During each workshop, participants are asked to look at work-life integration by identifying areas of their life (mental, emotional, spiritual and physical) where they need to dedicate more time or focus to mitigating stress, taking back control of their lives and preventing burnout.

Stephen Covey articulated how important it is to take back power and control in your own life. You can do this by getting clear on three things:

1. What you're most concerned about
2. What decisions you can influence
3. Most importantly, what decisions you have the complete power to action

For example, every single day you accept what you cannot change (e.g., the weather), but you change the way you respond to, in this case, the weather (e.g., umbrella, winter boots, sunhat, etc.). You choose to spend your time and energy only on those things that you can honestly influence or action.

Another revealing exercise that helps make work-life boundaries crystal clear is to write out a twenty-four-hour schedule of how you spend a typical day — classifying your time into specific categories. (See the Work-Life Integration Dinner Plate Activity on next page). What most people find is that without clear boundaries they readily give up the vital mental health boosters like play, connecting with family time and important "me" downtime — which are key to mitigating stress. I recall a female executive in her early forties, married with two children, coming up to speak with me after completing this exercise. With tears welling in her eyes she said,

"Catherine, I'm failing miserably at life right now. This exercise was painful to complete because other than squeezing in supper, a walk, bath, play and bedtime with my kids, my whole day is focused on outcomes. And I haven't had a good night's sleep in years. I'm crashing. I have no oxygen mask. I need help. I can't live this way one second longer."

Sometimes it just takes time to be accountable for your choices — taking back power and control — to realize that you're barely surviving. So, what's on your work-life integration plate today? Let's stop at the gift shop and pick up this important tool.

🎁 GIFT BOX RESILIENCY TOOLS

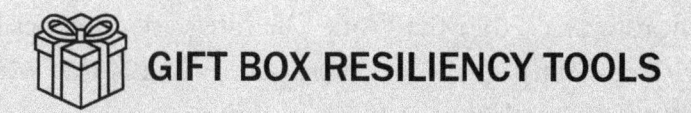

Work-life Integration Dinner Plate Activity

The goal of this exercise is to make you aware of how you divide up your time on a typical day (downloadable at www.catherineclarkconnects.com). Write down what a typical day would constitute for you using a twenty-four-hour clock, hour by hour. When do you usually get up and go to bed? Label your time blocks with one of the seven time categories, such as focus time vs. downtime. Although scrolling through social media can constitute downtime/playtime for some, I challenge you to focus on activities that do not involve screen time. Add up the hours in each category to reveal where you are missing key activities and where you are over-indulging.

Below you will find the time categories we all require:

Playtime	Time spent being spontaneous or creative, playfully engaged in experiences we enjoy. Anything that nurtures your soul like painting, playing with a pet, dancing or singing.	Hours per day

Connecting time	Time spent connecting with other people, ideally in person. Appreciating the connection and relationship we have with this person/people.	
Physical time	Time spent moving our bodies and engaged in exercise. Walking, cycling, swimming, indoor gym or outdoor individual/team sports.	
Mealtime	Time spent preparing and sitting down to enjoy a meal on your own or with family.	
Downtime	Time spent quietly reflecting, focusing on our feelings or simply doing nothing. Twenty minutes of mindfulness in the morning, relaxing without any specific goal.	
Sleep time	Time spent giving our brain and body the restorative rest they need. An essential time to consolidate learning, process and recover from the experiences of the day.	
Focus time	Time spent focusing on tasks in a goal-oriented way. Managing challenges that move us closer to achieving work, household and professional goals, for instance, grocery shopping and laundry.	

Is your plate balanced with healthy helpings of exercise, play, and connecting with friends/loved ones? Or do you find yourself bogged down in focused time? You're working so hard to complete tasks that you end up saying, "I can't possibly fit in lunch with my friend or a bike ride today." A work-life integration plan ensures that your plate has room for all the essential ingredients necessary for overall health and well-being. What's one small change that you can make today — one thing to start or stop doing?

BOUNDARIES 101

I bet that dinner plate exercise made you realize that you need to build some boundaries — emotional and physical — into your twenty-four-hour schedule. We do not place enough value on the benefits of setting healthy boundaries. But without them, we can end up sabotaging relationships, becoming resentful and getting burned out. And you'll keep finding yourself pushed down and stuck in the same dark box until you finally say enough is enough!

Setting clear boundaries is not about being selfish, it's being "self-full" (having self-love and self-respect to do what is best for you). It's learning to be a resiliency guru — putting your big rocks first — taking loving care of beautiful YOU. A resilient person, even facing the worst situation, can adopt a problem-solving attitude and clearly identify possible next steps. They know when not to respond to a seemingly urgent need in the outside world.

The thing is most of us never learned how to say no — especially those of us from the people-pleasing academy. So, you say "yes" way too often, fulfilling superhuman demands until you're flat-out exhausted. I watched my own mother selflessly do this for years. I followed in her footsteps becoming a professional "do for others," superhero mom and wife.

In his book, *Not Nice: Stop People Pleasing, Staying Silent & Feeling Guilty*, social confidence expert, Dr. Aziz Gazipura, uncovers the phenomenon he calls the "niceness cage" where faulty programming such as, "If I please others… then others will like me, love me, shower me with everything I want," keeps you stuck in a cycle of constantly seeking outside validation.[42] It's a dangerous thing indeed when our self-worth is tied to how others perceive or treat us. Rather than being an authentic expression of ourselves, being nice all the time is actually fear-based conditioning, preventing us from being vulnerable and opening up our dark package for others to see. Do you recognize yourself in this programming?

Glennon Doyle, in her book *Untamed*, talks about the need to free your inner cheetah from its cage by asking, "What do I really want as opposed to what does the world want from me?"[43] Good question. So, I'd suggest you go out and disappoint as many people as you want, as long as you're being truthful about your own needs. Remember, if you don't put your own oxygen mask on first, you're going to pass out on that plane, leaving you unable to help your kids, support your colleagues or even be around to feed your poor dog.

I usually only see a few hands go up in the air when I ask who's good at setting boundaries, yet the sheer volume of demands on time and energy today means that you have no other choice than to draw your line in the sand. "Self-stand" is my new buzz word for becoming what psychotherapist Terri Cole calls a "Boundary Boss," in her recent book by the same name. Cole created a "Boundary Boss Bill of Rights," to determine who has the privilege of being in your life, to make mistakes and to prioritize your own self-care without feeling guilty.[44] Many of my clients would be given a failing grade on this determination. Boundary-setting is an uber difficult skill, it can feel like a foreign language at first. But, with small steps and practice, you will become more empowered in all your relationships, especially the one you have with yourself.

Let's keep going and pick up a couple more boundary-setting tools at the gift shop.

GIFT BOX RESILIENCY TOOLS

Three essential practices for getting back on the road to setting healthy boundaries are:

- **VISUALIZATION** — Think of a specific situation where you currently feel disrespected and very conflicted. When it's safe to do so, close your eyes and visualize yourself confidently speaking up and asking for a change in behaviour. Use the formula: "When this happens (say situation), I feel (name the emotion). I would appreciate it if next time (ask for a specific actionable change)." Visualize and experience the feeling of being open, honest and proud of standing up for yourself. Breathe and smile.

- **PRACTISE AUTHENTICITY** — Each morning, spend a couple minutes looking in the mirror and practise telling yourself the authentic truth about the things you have minimized, glossed over or said "yes" to when you wanted to say "no." No more sugar-coating. For example, you could say, "If I'm really honest, I'm making excuses for (*friend's name*) disrespectful behaviour and I did or said (*say situation aloud*) to avoid conflict. I am playing small by telling white lies to (*friend's name)* instead of communicating what I really want and need. Today, I will be honest with myself and share my feelings with others about _____."

- **REACH OUT FOR HELP** — Connect with a trusted friend or therapist to practise putting these new boundaries into action.

SELF-CARE IS CRITICAL

> *"Your job is to fill your own cup, so it overflows. Then you can serve others, joyfully, from your saucer."*
> — Lisa Nichols

What I've learned from both my clients and my own work is that taking care of yourself is your number one priority. Giving yourself everything you need first — from that sun-soaked walk by the river, to alone time spent nurturing you and doing absolutely nothing — is vital to building true mental health resiliency. Whatever self-care is to you — do that. Self-care is imperative in order to live life with greater joy and ease — to actualize work-life integration.

When asked the question, "Do you take care of yourself?" most of my clients will answer yes — and even think, "What kind of question is that? Of course, I care about myself." When asked, "In what ways do you take care of yourself?" Well, that's where the pregnant pause happens.

What's your answer? For many of us, the phrase "self-care" just isn't in our personal lexicon. It's usually something like, "When I'm so dead-tired that I can't move off the couch, I just fall asleep there watching TV instead of cleaning up the kitchen." Now that's a sad state indeed!

What really constitutes self-care?

It's anything that we do deliberately in order to take care of our mental, emotional, spiritual and physical health. Self-care is remembering to stop at the gas station to make sure your tank is full and your four tires are topped up with air so you're roadworthy. Even though it's a simple concept in theory, it's easily overlooked and not viewed as critical. Yet good self-care has been proven to significantly improve mood and reduce anxiety. Building a caring relationship with yourself is the foundation for building an affirming relationship with anyone else.

Simply put, self-care can lead to genuine self-love. That's where a dark gift can be an important catalyst. Often our truest sense of self is only revealed when we're in the midst of a crisis — when we muster up the Herculean strength to get back up again. When we can say, "I'm so proud of myself — I just overcame a seemingly insurmountable obstacle. Now, I'm really deserving of celebration, pampering and self-renewal." We will explore this concept of self-love and how to nurture it more fully at Checkpoint 9.

Self-care might be something that you need to schedule in your calendar in order to nourish yourself regularly. Don't wait until you have a dark package delivery because even the smallest of self-care initiatives can bolster resiliency and prevent a downward spiral in the first place.

It's up to each of us to determine what self-care activities are affirming and healing. Nobody can do that for you. What soothes your soul and makes you feel cared for? Maybe it's a lazy Sunday morning, a long walk through the woods, baking bread or spending time alone in your bedroom playing the guitar. I challenge you to find new ways to take good care of yourself — be the top priority on your "to do" list. Carve self-care into your daily life with specific reminders in your cell phone or computer calendar. Or maybe you need to scrap that "to do" list all together and sink into simply being. Let go. Perhaps self-care doesn't require a "to do" list — a computer — a reminder. Maybe it's just embracing you beyond any kind of schedule. That's a hard concept I need to keep practising myself as a self-proclaimed over-scheduler.

In the end, do whatever feels easy and brings you joy. Be mindful and unapologetic about your self-care non-negotiables. Make people aware that you have a "hard stop" on your own time.

☕ COFFEE WITH CATHERINE

As we sip our coffee, let's ponder your use of time for loving self-care:

1. **Make a list of your current commitments and activities.** For each commitment, ask yourself, "Am I consciously choosing it? Is it my responsibility? How important is it to me? How much pleasure do I get from it?"
2. **Where are your biggest time vampires or time suckers?** What do you need to change to claim this time back (e.g., delegate to employee/family member, productivity app, turn sounds off on your devices, uninterrupted time blocking, saying "no")?
3. **Do you have a "transition ritual"** that helps you change gears from focus time (work) to personal or playtime? For example, at 5 p.m., play your favourite song, have a dance party, change your outfit, make a list of the top three things you need to do the next day, then close the book. Make it harder to go back to work after hours by logging out of all work programs at the end of the day or fully shutting down your computer.
4. **In order to align your daily tasks to your key priorities ("big rocks"),** what changes do you need to make? What do you need to do less of and what do you need to do more of to realize work-life integration?

🎁 GIFT BOX RESILIENCY TOOLS

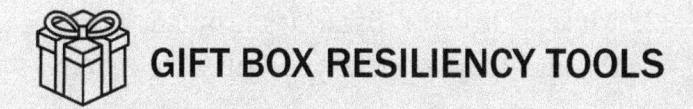

Self-care Plan/Checklist

We do not want to make self-care feel like one more thing on your "to do" list or a chore. Nonetheless, I'd suggest that you set up a fourteen-day self-care routine and track how you feel before and after. Remember that self-care may seem like a foreign language now, but with practice it will become second nature.

Let's revisit your priorities list to identify what needs to be added into your self-care plan and what needs to be eliminated. Communicate your needs to family/friends, ask for their input and schedule those things in your agenda today. Or try simply being in the moment with whatever is happening. During the next week, make a list of the things that cause you to feel like your best, most focused and healthy self ("I'm doing something I love!"). Also note down what makes you feel miserable, resentful or scattered ("I'm doing something I loathe!"). The more specific you can be, the better. Having made informed choices, you can now set up your self-care routine as follows:

1. Create a "hell no" list, with things you know you don't like, or you no longer want to do (things you dread, loathe or feel drained by).

2. Make a "hell yes" list (things you are looking forward to, that make you feel energized and magnetic).

3. Create a healthy and nutritious menu for the week, a shopping list and a cooking schedule for each night. Delegate if possible. Sit down and mindfully consume your meals.

4. Make sleep a priority and read up about good sleep hygiene. Adults usually need seven to eight hours of sleep each night. Be consistent. Go to bed at the same time each night and get up at the same time each morning. Turn off screens ninety minutes before you want to fall asleep, have a dark, cool bedroom and bedtime ritual (tea, read, bath).

5. Exercise to increase your serotonin levels, which leads to improved mood and energy. Choose a form of exercise that you like and make it fun — pump up the volume and dance in the kitchen!

6. Follow-up with your medical and/or holistic health care appointments. Checkups are a form of prevention-focused self-care.

7. Spend quality time with loved ones. Family games night or dinner with a friend.

8. Schedule daily relaxation exercises and/or practise mindfulness meditation. Make it easy and get an app on your cell phone like Insight Timer or Headspace.

9. Give yourself time to do nothing at all or at least one relaxing activity. Make sure that you have downtime. Block it in your schedule so that you actually follow through with it.

10. Do at least one pleasurable activity (playtime) every day.

11. Look for opportunities to laugh — a really big belly laugh!

Now that we have self-care and a healthy dose of self-discipline in our front seat, let's gas up and continue on the roadway. We're going to get very good at embracing all kinds of change in our lives — especially the unwanted ones — at the next checkpoint.

"Imagine the person you'd become if you stopped trying to fix others and put that energy into yourself!"
— Florence Given, *Women Don't Owe You Pretty*

CHECKPOINT 7

Challenging Change

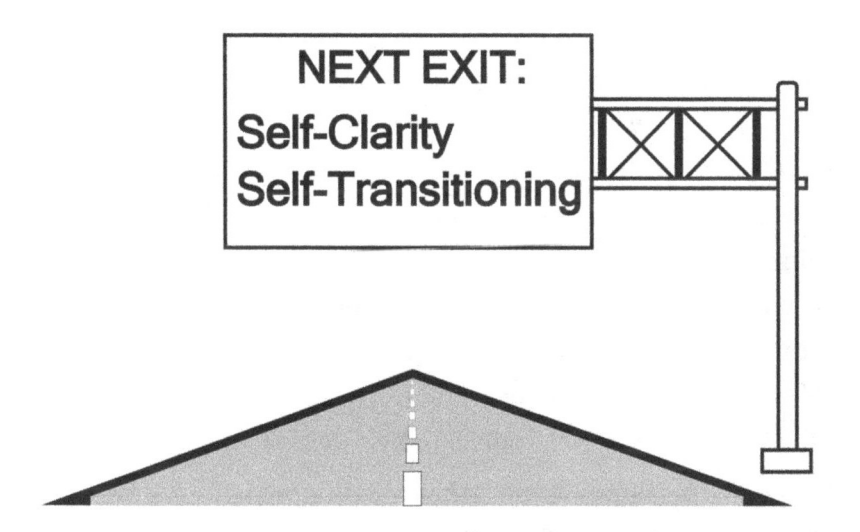

"It is not the strongest of the species that survives, nor the most intelligent, but the one most responsive to change."
— Charles Darwin

"What we call obstacles are really the way the world and our entire experience teach us where we're stuck."
— Pema Chödrön

If change is happening every second of every day, why do so many of us shudder at the thought of it, instead of seeing it as an opportunity for growth? As human beings, we can get very set in our ways. We certainly don't want the kind of uncomfortable change a dark package can bring. We'd rather bury our head under the covers and hope that it will all go away.

I've facilitated many workshops on managing change and when I ask participants to complete the sentence, "Change makes me feel _____," the responses always range from "scared" to "excited — bring it on!" I suspect you're here at this highway exit because you're ready to embrace the idea that change can be good. I'm so glad you're open to this viewpoint.

You're willing to look at change as an opportunity for your soul's evolution — a brilliantly disguised dark gift.

According to the Greek philosopher Heraclitus, "The only thing that is constant is change." What I think he meant by this statement was that change is the fundamental nature of reality — it can't be resisted — but we can learn to live in harmony with it. We can learn to fully embrace it.

So, if we view self-transitioning more like a river that flows with a steady, slow current, as well as the swirling, wild rapids — we might enjoy the entire boat ride of life a little bit more. Or, as Heraclitus suggests, we might learn to "just go with the flow" instead of fighting against it. In doing so, we can welcome new beginnings like the Spring Equinox and see the beauty in endings like the tapestry of burnt orange and red maple trees in the fall.

When we stop struggling with our challenging changes, we can make peace with our "former self." We can let go and put into practice the self-surrender strategies that we added to our toolkit at Checkpoint 5.

We can learn to trust that, like the tree stripped of its leaves in fall, our soil is being nourished by change — we're putting down new roots for our rebirth.

Life changes strengthen our resiliency and edge us closer to self-fulfillment. As we learned at Checkpoint 4, transitions are made easier when we accept that much of what happens to us is not within our power and control anyway. Yet, with self-clarity we can choose to act only on those things that are worth our time, energy and effort — and let go of all the rest. Or, when adversity forces us into uncomfortable, uncharted territory, we can recite our own version of the well-known *Serenity Prayer*: *"God, grant me the serenity to accept the things I cannot change, the courage to change the things I can, and wisdom to know the difference."* Only the last line could read: *"The wisdom to hide all the bodies of the people who pissed me off,"* if you're one of my dark humour friends because sometimes it's a dark sense of humour that can help us navigate difficult life changes.

CAREER CHANGE

> *"Sometimes when one bridge is burning, the bright light illuminates a whole new bridge on the horizon."*
> — Catherine Clark

One of the most destabilizing changes that many of us will face in our lives is job loss and unemployment. As a career counsellor, I see the pain and despair that is handed to clients all the time in the form of layoff notices, being fired, or simply needing to resign because a company's values are no longer congruent with your own.

Regardless of whether an employee saw it coming or it came as a complete surprise, the reaction is almost always one of shock, anger and fear. This reaction is a very dark package that is almost never immediately seen as a "blessing in disguise."

Job loss does, however, offer up the opportunity to rise above adversity. For those who are willing to suspend judgement and face their fears, it can be an incredible way to pivot. It can be a *chance* to move in a new direction. For example, to retrain in a new, more fulfilling career — in an industry you absolutely love — that aligns with your core values. This pivot is entirely possible with the right mindset, support and counselling services needed to relaunch yourself.

Most large organizations and government agencies provide outplacement services, which help employees with career counselling and job search strategies. But, there's only one way to navigate this change and that's to go through the uncomfortable process of it. If we do not turn toward this painful change, we remain stuck — the pain owns us.

In 2008, the Global Financial Crisis sent shock waves across North America. Gary, a big, burly man in his early forties, found himself in my office, fidgeting in his chair like a snake trying desperately to shed its skin. This visit was the first time that he had ever set foot in a counselling agency. There was no hiding his complete and total discomfort — his eyes darting back and forth in rhythm to his shaking knee. I nodded reassuringly as he lamented,

"My job's never coming back. What can I possibly do for work now? I'm done!"

Due to the recession, Gary was laid off from his high-paying job of twenty years — working on the assembly line for an automotive parts manufacturer. And he was right — his job wasn't coming back any time soon. He was terrified. Little did he know at the time that this layoff would be his greatest gift. He would qualify for a government program to go back to school and retrain to become a veterinary technician. His lifelong passion for working with animals would be turned into a rewarding career, one he never would have pursued had he not been taken out of a comfortable job with great benefits.

More than anything, career transitions are an incredible vehicle to gain self-clarity and to master self-transitioning. They help us address inner blocks, uncover existing strengths, build self-esteem and pinpoint careers that are a much better match for our personality, learning style and passions. Job loss is the "off" button that gets forcibly pushed. It's because of the pause that a myriad of life reboots are made possible.

It's the deep existential "pain of it" that becomes the "gain of it."

When you're suddenly unemployed, you must take stock of how you spend your precious time, what truly matters, and come face to face with the parts of yourself that you left behind — your hopes and dreams tucked away in an abandoned childhood box.

This transformation is why career counselling is some of the most rewarding work I do, especially with young high school students who are the most open and receptive to change. It's a joy to witness the "A-ha!" moment when a student discovers something they're passionate about. Students like Leo, who set his sights on being a theatre set designer, even though his parents were fixated on him becoming an electrical engineer.

I'll never forget how we brainstormed a plan for Leo to pay for the theatre program that his parents were not willing to help finance. His eyes shone like headlights when he turned to me and said, *"You mean I could take a short certificate course to work as a drill operator and make the money needed to pay for the stage designer/props program myself?"* Leo had found a way to take his love of working with tools and heavy equipment to train for a job that would later finance his true career aspiration. He had found a work-around for his parents' inflexible mindset in order to take control of his education decision-making.

Let's face it — the future world of work will involve lots of self-transitioning by doing multiple jobs, being self-employed and trying a variety of careers. So, we might as well embrace it. I've had so many different jobs in this lifetime I've lost count. My latest course correction is something that I have loved to do all my life but never made space to do — writing.

At the very least, I suggest you do something you love that's congruent with your personal values, whether you're just starting out or you're suddenly unemployed. And try to do one really unique job that will always make people laugh at a dinner party or get an interviewer's attention. No one ever tires of hearing my funny *I Love Lucy*-style stories of flying pickles and olive jars crashing off the conveyor belt at my pickle factory summer job.

Let's stop for coffee now and look at teachable moments — times in our life when we can pause, reflect and course correct.

☕ COFFEE WITH CATHERINE

While we sip our coffee, here are some career coaching questions that I would typically ask to help you get unstuck, uncover your passions and consider new career directions:

1. What has the latest adversity in your life — such as a job loss or forced career change — taught you about yourself? What's one good thing?

2. What could you do for hours on end and never get bored? It could be something you did as a child, for a hobby or as part of a previous job.
3. What did you play with as a child or love to do? Even if you had a difficult childhood, you might have loved reading, soccer or playing piano.
4. What could you talk about for hours on end that lights you up? (Don't even get me started on human motivation and personality theory.)
5. If you were independently wealthy, what would you do with your time? Where would you live? What would a typical day look like?
6. After you die, what are the three things that you want to be remembered for?
7. How do you know when you're swimming with the current? What's easy, enjoyable, meaningful and fulfilling for you? For example, I like freedom, variety and autonomy in my work. Coaching, talking, writing and presenting do not feel like work to me.
8. What feels like a waste of your time and drains you? Perhaps it's commuting to work, but working from home has solved this issue for you?

Act now:
1. Grab your journal. Answer the questions above. Start first by writing a list of at least ten things you're grateful for right now. Set an intention

with a specific date and time for when you would like to be working in the career you're passionate about.
2. Do some "act as if" future self-journalling and write about your first day, week, month in the job of your dreams with as much vivid detail as possible. Close your eyes and really feel the emotions.
3. Do online research to identify professionals to contact. Then reverse engineer it. Take one action step every day (i.e., information interviewing) to move toward your career change goal. Solicit the help and support of your tribe and/or career counsellor.

GIFT BOX RESILIENCY TOOLS

Core Values Exercise

Change can shock your system and disrupt your preconceived notion about what really matters in your life. It brings to light what no longer serves you. The gift is the "Aha" moment when you finally align your actions to your newfound values. Please complete the exercise on the next page to uncover and reinforce the values and non-negotiables in your resiliency toolkit:

1. Make a list of the top ten values in your life right now (e.g., love, freedom, learning, health, loyalty, adventure, fun, creativity, respect, solitude, community, beauty, etc.). Google "values exercise" if you need to find a full list to ponder.

2. Rank these values from one to ten.

3. Evaluate each value. How important is this value for me right now on a scale from one to ten?

4. Modify your list, if necessary, and pick your top five values.

5. Compare your current activities and career against your list of values. How are you fulfilling each value? What do you need to tweak or do differently?

BRIDGING CHANGE

> *"When we are no longer able to change a situation, we are challenged to change ourselves."*
> — Viktor Frankl

Let's break this whole idea of self-transitioning down a little bit more. Now that we're at this exit, we might as well understand the psychological process of change. William Bridges, PhD developed and first published the Bridges Transition Model in his 1991 book, *Managing Transitions: Making the Most of Change*, which has since become the gold standard of how to understand change and process transitions.

"Change is simply a single event, a "happening" or a moment in time. And tomorrow the change will be yesterday's news. Whereas, transition is the psychological process we must go through to fully embrace and live the change."[45]

So, let's normalize the internal, psychological transition that unfolds when any change or a dark gift lands on your doorstep, whether that's getting laid off at work, a car accident or being diagnosed with cancer. Bridges identified three distinct stages of transition to attain greater self-awareness:

1. *Firstly, every transition starts with an **Ending**.*

    Paradoxical but true. This first phase of transition begins when people identify what they are losing and learn how to manage that loss. In March 2020, our lives as socializers, world-travellers, theatregoers, live sport-watchers, café-lovers and family holiday-celebrators were put on hold. This change was a profound change that required us to leave behind our former way of life.

2. *The second stage of transition can only come after the letting go or grieving stage is completed and is called the **Neutral Zone**.*

> The in-between stage where the old is gone but the new isn't fully active. This stage is like being right smack in the middle of the second or third Covid-19 lockdown wondering what the new rules of engagement are. We might know our old way of life is no longer possible, but we don't yet have a roadmap of the "new normal." It's a critical psychological realignment stage, which frustratingly trips many of us up. This destabilization is often a good reason to reach out for mental health support and the comfort of friends and community.

3. *The last stage is **Beginnings**, which means we embrace a new way to look at the world, see possibilities and adjust our attitudes.*

> Beginnings mean we start investing our energy in a new direction, new mindset and a new way of being in the world. Keeping with the Covid-19 example, the beginning phase could be a small backyard gathering as the new normal, instead of a large house party.

As you can see, transitioning became a very common theme during the global pandemic from 2020 onwards. And it will continue to be at the forefront for the next decade. So, we might as well practise getting good at change. Thankfully, most people are able to successfully transition through any change once they are able to find the calm in the chaos. They find a way to invest new energy in hope for a better tomorrow. Without hope — belief in a brighter bridge ahead — we are merely surviving.

On our mental health resiliency road trip, those "new beginnings" are waiting for us — straight ahead on the wide-open road. We just need to put our car back in drive and leave the "doom and gloom," bad news stories and pity parties behind. So, let's practise by stopping at the gift shop to pick up more self-transitioning strategies.

Top Ten Self-Transitioning Strategies
Here's a list of strategies that help you flex your resiliency muscle to keep your mental health in check when a traumatic change is happening.

1. **Take some time to let yourself fully grieve** — We've all experienced grief for what life was like pre-Covid, for example. Fully acknowledge this trauma and write it down, then reflect on the pros and cons of each of these changes. Remind yourself of what has remained stable and comfortable — express gratitude for these small blessings.

2. **Embrace all your emotions** — Breathe, check in with yourself, notice what you're experiencing: volatility, shaking, sweating, a pit in your stomach, hopelessness, headaches, insomnia, inability to think clearly or any other symptoms. What if you reframed your fear or anger? Using your skills from Checkpoint 2, try to look at your situation from a different perspective.

3. **Be kind and loving to yourself, especially if you're anxious or depressed** — Show up for yourself every day — do one little loving thing. Review your self-care plan from Checkpoint 6. Say to yourself, "I'm doing better today than

last month or last year." Or maybe you feel crappy — that's okay too. Growth, like grief, is not a straight line — it's a flowing river and there are rapids ahead. Like Heraclitus, just go with the flow — surrender.

4. **Take mini breaks from everything** — Rest your mind. Turn off the newsfeed. Stop thinking so much. Make room for playtime and downtime. Meditate. Practise the mindfulness strategies in Checkpoint 5.

5. **Remind yourself of your "big picture" goals** — Make a vision board of all the places and things you plan to do in your life. Hang it on a wall where you will see it and smile every day. Dream. Stay optimistic by saying, "When one door closes, another one opens."

6. **Create new rituals** — A bedtime and morning routine as suggested in Checkpoint 5 would help immensely. Let go of the old and make a list of new holidays to celebrate online or in person with family/friends, get dressed up, make a special dinner or host a family games night.

7. **Prepare an "if ever" action plan** — Draft up an emergency call list, what to take with you in an evacuation, important documents, passwords, including where to find them, and things you want a loved one to know should something suddenly change. Once you have completed this plan, keep it somewhere safe and secure in case you need it in the future. Peace of mind is the only goal of this exercise.

8. **Marvel at your resiliency muscles** — Remind yourself of a time when you've bounced back successfully. What did you do then that you can keep applying to this change? Practise that one doable action today. Keep taking deep breaths.

9. **Say good-bye to the pity party** — Guilt, shame and hopelessness may have been your comfortable friends for a long time. It's hard to say goodbye to long-time friends, but it starts with a new self-belief that we will reinforce at Checkpoint 10.

10. **Reach out for help** — Withdrawing from your life altogether, being a lone wolf, or constantly struggling to figure things out takes a toll on your mental and physical health. If your heart feels heavy, share your burden with trusted friends and reach out to a mental health professional. See the mental health supports listed at www.catherineclarkconnects.com.

TRAUMATIC CHANGE

"We can create a narrative in which trauma is seen as a fork in the road that enhances the appreciation of paradox — loss and gain, grief and gratitude, vulnerability and strength."
— Dr. Martin E.P. Seligman

Just like a butterfly emerging from a chrysalis, traumatic change is often the difficult catalyst that we need to realize our amazing potential. Even if it's the last thing we'd put on our wish list. I'm not suggesting that we actively seek out hardships, but taking risks and facing your fears almost always delivers mammoth post-traumatic growth. I wouldn't be stretching my capacities to author this book, had I not faced my own mortality or had life-altering experiences.

Dr. Kanako Taku, professor at Oakland University, researched hundreds of traumatic events, in particular those that challenge a person's core beliefs and contribute to mental disorders (e.g., PTSD, depression) and found they are, indeed, some of the greatest contributors to post-traumatic growth. But it's also the smaller repeated struggles or more ordinary adversities we take for granted — such as caring for a parent who is suddenly diagnosed with Alzheimer's, changing schools or being in a psychologically-draining relationship — that can provide important opportunities for growth. What's essential to keep in mind is that post-traumatic growth is not a direct result of trauma, but rather how we psychologically transition through the traumatic change. As positive psychologists Dr. Richard G. Tedeschi and Dr. Lawrence Calhoun explain, "Someone who is already resilient when trauma occurs won't experience PTG because a resilient person isn't rocked to the core by an event and doesn't have to seek a new belief system."[46] Now that's the bounce-forward muscle we're going for here.

So, let's just agree that hardships and traumatic life changes give us the opportunity to better understand ourselves, our worldview and our relationships. Perhaps more than anything else they literally propel us toward new future life intentions. It may take great courage to get to the other side of this struggle. Some days, that courage may simply involve getting out of bed in the morning. But persistence and perseverance after repeated falls, demonstrate your extraordinary capacity to rise. They reinforce the importance of building up a toolkit brimming with personal mental health resources that's always at the ready.

Here's a traumatic story from my stock of personal hardships that infused my toolkit with a myriad of coping resources and changed my mindset. It's also a really good example of transitioning through the psychological struggle from feeling everything's "Impossible" to rewriting the word to spell "I'm possible." I still draw upon these tools and adaptive coping strategies today.

Can you imagine going through a pregnancy with a broken leg? I can sense you furrowing your brow just imagining that kind of pain. Just so you know, this break could only be repaired with surgery, but that wasn't possible until after delivery. So, you're probably wondering, "How the heck did she do that? Did she get in a car accident while newly pregnant?" Actually, the car accident that crushed my leg and landed me in a cast, requiring multiple surgeries, happened fourteen months prior. That's right, I became pregnant with a cast on my very broken leg. I even received kudos from my orthopaedic surgeon for having that kind of libido!

The freak car accident that changed my life forever happened when my son was not quite a year old. I went from being an active new mom to an immobilized new mom in a wheelchair.

When tragedy strikes you can really wallow in the "ending," unable to see any positives.

I kept asking, "Why me? Why did I have to drive to work that day when I was feeling so sick and comatose with no reflexes at all?" When the parking lot machine ticket was too hard to reach, "Why didn't I just take a moment to put the car in park before opening the car door and pivoting, stretching my entire left side toward the ticket machine?" I can still feel the seething burn of metal and concrete against bone as my right foot slipped off the brake and my left leg was crushed. The piercing sounded like a runaway train screeching to a halt on the tracks. The gush of blood poured from my ragdoll limb before I realized that I had to put the car in park. But the damage had been done. You can never go back through a door that's been slammed shut behind you.

So, if someone had said to me, "Catherine, you're going to almost lose your leg in a car accident, then you'll go through an entire pregnancy with a broken leg," I'd have said there's no way. "And then you're going to give birth to a baby girl, need surgery again and be on crutches in rehabilitation for another two years. You'll feel powerless and deeply depressed — immobilized." I'd have said, "Please, no. Haven't I had enough?"

In all honesty, I was ready to give up, but being a mom propels you forward — it's like a perseverance turbo booster. I had no other choice than to transition from the old version of myself to embracing a new, physically challenged Catherine.

I was drowning in the middle of Bridge's neutral stage when it dawned on me: "Physically challenged people have babies too." I could sleep on the futon, so I never have to climb the stairs, and I could push my baby around in a bassinet on wheels with my crutches. I could use a transfer board to slide her down from the bassinet for nursing. Short of giving her a bath, I would be able to manage my own care and hers too — all on my own. Deep inside me, a switch of hopefulness and empowerment was flicked on.

So began my transition into the "new beginnings" stage of change. A self-clarity like never before. I found so much to be grateful for, as I cuddled my angel daughter for hours, gazing deeply into her eyes with profound love. I promised her that we would be strong, resilient women together, forever — realizing the beauty in our dark packages. She remains one of my greatest blessings — born out of adversity. This life-changing adversity was the route to my true hidden superpower — gritty, resolute perseverance.

GRIT AND GROWTH MINDSET

> *"Being gritty doesn't mean not showing pain or pretending everything is O.K. in the face of a difficult change. In fact, when you look at healthy, successful people, they are very self-aware or extraordinarily meta-cognitive. They're able to say things like, "Dude, I totally lost my temper this morning." That ability to reflect on yourself is a signature of grit."*
> — Dr. Angela Duckworth

Psychologist Dr. Angela Duckworth coined the idea of "grit" to describe people who have a growth mindset and are highly resilient in the face of life's challenges. Being gritty is being able to push yourself through difficult circumstances, finding a way above, below or around an obstacle, temporarily failing while consistently moving toward a passionate goal. If the key attribute of a resilient person is optimism, then the salient attribute of a gritty person is a sustained "never give up" effort toward achieving a goal. We sure as heck need more grit when the time comes to embrace our dark packages and have grace under fire.

Dr. Duckworth describes "grit" as the engine that moves us toward a goal, while resilience is the oil for the engine.[47]

Can we learn to be grittier?

The good news is that although some people are born grittier than others, experience is the best teacher. You can learn to be gritty just by being open to experiences, maintaining a curious mind and staying on a difficult course to see where it will lead you — remaining in that tough job just a bit longer, finishing your last semester of university, and getting through your last round of chemotherapy. At this checkpoint, I want you to think about how gritty you already are in the face of change. Let's look under your hood again to see whether you have more of a growth versus a fixed mindset.

Growth Versus Fixed Mindset
A person can't have grit without first acquiring a growth mindset, which Dr. Carol Dweck identified as "believing that your basic qualities are things you can cultivate through your efforts."[48] The characteristics of a fixed versus a growth mindset may be summarized as follows:

With a fixed mindset, you:
- Believe your qualities (e.g., IQ) are innate and carved in stone
- Think success should come easily if you're smart or talented
- Tend to give up in the face of setbacks or failure

With a growth mindset, you:
- Believe success comes from perseverance and effort
- See failure and criticism as an opportunity for growth
- Learn and grow from change by accepting it
- Embrace challenges

According to Dr. Dweck, these mindsets exist on a continuum and are influenced by our cultural background. You can have a fixed mindset in one area (e.g., mathematical concepts) but a growth mindset in another (e.g., seeking out networking opportunities).

Adopting a growth mindset means putting in effort rather than relying on our previous ability. If we want to adapt to whatever change is thrown at us, we need to keep building our grittiness. Simply thinking about a growth mindset can apparently make you more open to developing a grittier way of operating in the world. So, go out and think gritty thoughts.

Let's stop at the gift shop now and dig a little deeper into our grittiness.

GIFT BOX RESILIENCY TOOLS

Grit and growth mindsets change over time and are influenced by our thoughts, beliefs, experiences and practices. Here are a few ways to learn how to build this mindset:

1. Interview someone who has experienced a tragedy and lived to tell the tale — what helped them through it?

2. Find examples of grit in nature. Think about how you can be more like a tulip bulb or a tree sprouting in the rubble of a junkyard.

3. Embrace mistakes as temporary setbacks and opportunities to grow and change.

4. Everything is "figureoutable" if you break a problem down into bite-sized, manageable pieces and set realistic goals. Reverse-engineer your goals.

5. Heraclitus said, "The only constant in life is change." Sometimes a goal needs to be abandoned because it is no longer attainable. Practise self-compassion. Say the *Serenity Prayer* and fully surrender.

6. Create a goal that is just outside of your reach. Finish it. Keep doing this until you can reach any goal you set your mind to. Dr. Duckworth calls this doing "the hard thing" exercise.

7. Try the "Grit Pie Problem" exercise. Think of a problem that you need to solve. Each slice of the pie is a cause of the overall "Pie Problem." Which causes do you have control over? What can you change? Eat those pieces first.

8. Practise observing how your mistakes can actually be really funny. Laugh at yourself at least three times today. Remember this will make a funny story one day.

What else makes some people so good at change?
We all have that friend who wouldn't hesitate to try bungee jumping, pivots quickly to a great new career after being downsized or turns a cancer diagnosis into a spiritual awakening. Why is that? Sometimes it comes down to your comfort level with change and your capacity for change.

Our capacity for change is affected by a variety of factors, including our upbringing, education, experience, attitude, access to information, level of trust, degree of involvement in the change and the timing of a change.

For example, I have been called in to support employees who were ambushed by a hostile corporate takeover where trust was completely broken. These employees demonstrated little capacity to cope, as they felt so powerless and overwhelmed. I've also supported employees who were informed well in advance of a probable merger and acquisition and how it might affect their job security. With open, honest communication, especially from senior management, the capacity of these employees to cope with drastic change was much higher. They were saying things like, "We can handle these changes — we'll be okay" versus feeling powerless.

What does your comfort level with change mean? It refers to how at ease we feel about a change and how we think it will affect our life — both at work and personally. The more positive experiences we've had with previous changes, the more likely we are to look at new experiences in a positive light. A person with a high comfort level might say, "I like change." These people are the change agents that we pointed out at the beginning of this checkpoint, who are the first to say, "Sign me up!" So, it stands to reason that having a high level of comfort and capacity for change would make you more resilient in the face of change.

High comfort + high capacity = ability to rock change and be curious about what happens next.

If you moved around a lot as a kid, you are more likely to have a higher curiosity quotient (discussed at Checkpoint 8) — that is, you enjoy and are open to new experiences. It usually also means you developed stronger self-clarity and self-transitioning skills at a young age — which only augments your capacity for change as an adult.

The good thing is that you can increase your capacity for change just by hanging out with people who are change agents. I call these people your expanders. They're the friends who are always trying new activities — the hang gliders and bungee jumpers — the ones who push you outside of your comfort zone. They're more willing to take risks, but also willing to learn from their mistakes. Or, borrowing from Theodore Roosevelt's famous speech, "They get in the arena!"

Believe me, these people are the ones that you want on your team. They ask questions, learn as much as they can about a specific change and remain open to the possibility that there will be a positive outcome. They're willing to adapt and remain hopeful in the face of adversity.

Gleaned from fifteen years of studying survivors of trauma, Dr. Martin E. P. Seligman, founder of positive psychology, identified the single most important trait for post-traumatic growth: learned optimism. He noted survivors with an optimistic attitude say things like, "I'm not giving up. This setback is temporary and changeable; it's just this one situation; and I can do something about it."[49] They're just better equipped to thrive despite adversity.

Perhaps the best antidote to traumatic change is "tragic optimism," a phrase coined by the existential-humanistic psychologist and Holocaust survivor Viktor Frankl. Tragic optimism refers to the ability to find meaning and purpose amid the inevitable tragedies of our human existence, instead of being crushed or overwhelmed by them.[50]

It's also a practical way to escape "learned helplessness" — that psychological predisposition to catastrophize and fixate on the "worst case scenario." The tragically optimistic keep going in the face of setbacks instead of giving up. They make space for learning, hope and meaning in both good and bad situations. It's like saying "yes" to the little moments that make life worth living — a sunset, the sound of rain, or a dog wagging its tail — despite pain and suffering.

To adopt this mindset we need to keep practising the reframing techniques we learned at Checkpoint 4 like reframing the stress of highway driving as a "challenge" rather than a threat to your survival. I'd also suggest you record "optimism" affirmations on your phone such as, "I've got this!" "I'm resilient," and, "I've learned to adapt to whatever life throws at me." It's so great when you can hear your own affirming voice. Repeat these affirmations every day so that they become second nature. Then, when it's time to get in the driver's seat, you'll have everything you need to have full control of the wheel.

Okay, it's time for a quick break — stretch, drink some water, jog on the spot to get the blood flowing — before we get back on the road. Give yourself a big pat on the back. You've come so far! Let's start our engines again and learn how to fully embrace the next unavoidable dark detour — death and profound grief.

> *"I've interviewed and portrayed people who've withstood some of the ugliest things life can throw at you, but the one quality all of them seem to share is an ability to maintain hope for a brighter morning — even during our darkest nights."*
> — Oprah Winfrey

CHECKPOINT 8

Living Through Loss

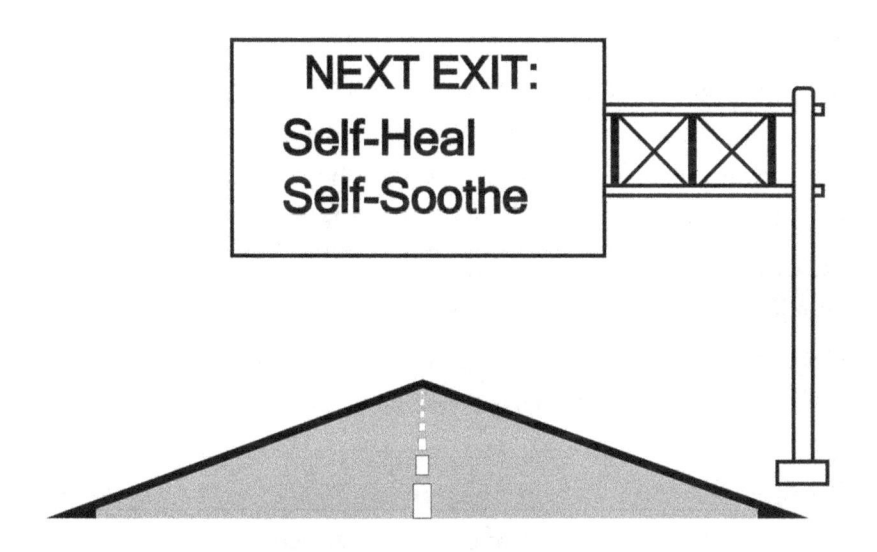

*"Your grief for what you've lost lifts a mirror
up to where you are bravely working."*
— Rumi

At Checkpoint 7, we learned that having a grit and a growth mindset will get you through the destabilizing changes and detours on the road to mental health resiliency. No one can completely avoid painful roadblocks, including grief. Although, I do wish we could skip this exit. But, as human beings, we must all experience loss — both the death of our loved ones and the erosion of our own minds and bodies. This dark package we're handed is universal — there's no avoiding it.

We have faith in many things — ourselves, others and the future. Yet, when someone we love dies, our faith and entire foundation can be shaken. It may seem like the world will never be the same again. We wonder if we'll ever feel better. I'm here to tell you, that it will get better, little by little.

You may also be wondering how could anything good possibly come from death and dying? There are benefits to grief. Grief is terrible — painful, raw and confusing. The truth is that grief has the capacity to profoundly transform us. Becoming more resilient, which means we are better able to cope with challenges later in life, is a common human response to loss. So, grief isn't all bad. Over time, it can change our perspective and how we view our world.

I don't believe time always heals — although often it does. Yet time does clear space so that our grief, pain and heartache can coexist with our new sense of self. We just need time to be in that dark place.

We need spaciousness to learn to let go and surrender to grief — to uncover authentic "gifts" that can emerge such as:

- Creating new connections
- Becoming more fully engaged in life
- Seeing things in a new and profound light

- Gratefulness — appreciating more of the present moment
- Becoming spiritually awake — aligning with a higher power source
- Self-knowing — the realization that you can heal yourself

Unfortunately, few people in our society look at grief as a transformative process. In fact, a plethora of societal beliefs and myths often hold us back from doing the work necessary to gain true insight. There isn't a Grief 101 subject in school, so how could we possibly be automatically good at it?

Even though I'm a trained professional with twenty-five years of experience, that doesn't mean I get to avoid the heavy lifting of grief. I'm thankful for my own heart-wrenching experiences. They've informed me and made me a stronger, better-equipped therapist. Because, after all, if you've lived a similar experience, you can more deeply connect with the same suffering in someone else and provide much-needed empathy.

At this Good Grief checkpoint, let's dispel some of the common stigmatizing phrases that keep us stuck in our grief. We've all been there, whether on the giving or receiving end of these words. You cringe when you hear yourself saying them or when they're mindlessly spoken to you. I'm referring to anything that's simply not true, or anything that openly encourages you to move away from grief instead of "leaning into" grief's full experience. I call these phrases platitudes that are unhelpful and damaging because grief is meant to be experienced in whatever way, or pace, is right for you, the griever.

Some of the platitudes that we often say to ourselves or to someone who has lost a loved one, can stop the grieving process in its tracks, namely:

- "I'm tough — I can't show any weakness." (self-stigma)
- "I need to pull myself together and get on with life." (self-stigma)
- "Be thankful he/she/they are no longer suffering." (societal stigma)
- "Be strong," or saying, "I'm fine," even when you're barely able to speak. (self-stigma)
- "At least he/she/they're not in pain any longer." (societal stigma)
- "Everything happens for a reason." (my most despised platitude)
- "Please do this mourning thing privately and as quickly as possible." (workplace stigma)

At this exit, I've put on my grief counsellor driving gloves so that I can be as supportive as possible. I also want to ensure that you have access to some tools that will lessen the sting of loss and create a clearing for greater self-insight. I've put more stories and additional resources in a "grief parking lot" in the downloadable resources kit at www.catherineclarkconnects.com to support some of our most difficult losses (e.g., euthanizing a pet, death by suicide and miscarriage).

At this checkpoint, let's investigate some of the hidden benefits in this dark package, as well as the grieving process, challenges and ways to cope. Then you'll have the option to visit the parking lot to go deeper into more specific grief situations, all with an eye toward gathering the tools needed for self-soothing, self-healing and post-traumatic growth. Maybe what you really need is to give yourself permission to be happy again, permission to live the kind of life that your deceased loved one would have wanted for you. Let's stay on that road together.

GIFTS OF GRIEF UNWRAPPED

"The gifts in grief are often hidden from view but larger than life in their expansiveness."
— Catherine Clark

Through my work as a trauma counsellor and my own life experiences, I've witnessed the capacity of the human spirit to persevere. I've seen how a team or community can come together through a shared experience of grief. The rebuilding that occurs, gives group members a sense of belonging, hope and peace. One of the hidden benefits that I've observed is a strengthening of trust as people begin to better understand the suffering of others. This trust leads to greater overall empathy as we learn how to be more sensitive and caring.

When I'm called into a company to help staff deal with a co-worker's death, my goal is to give people permission to openly grieve, heal and learn what to say to be more supportive. Providing early intervention in the form of group support, namely, critical incident stress debriefing (CISD), a heartfelt conversation or helping people gain access to individual support services — such as an employee assistance program (EAP) — is both compassionate and wise.

Picture this: Frank, a well-liked fifty-five-year-old corporate executive is suddenly killed in a small plane crash. His colleagues are grief-stricken. I'm called in to support the team in their grief, unpack emotions and normalize the experience of sudden loss. When there's no chance for a goodbye or final conversation, it makes the untimely death that much more difficult to accept.

I don't have a magic formula, but I can tell you that getting support as soon as possible after traumatic news can prevent a downward spiral and greatly facilitate the heavy lifting that is grief. In this situation, the team bonded together, shed tears, shared stories and planned a memory book and memorial for Frank. This sharing circle helped them move to a place of gratitude and appreciation for the lessons learned while in his presence, and the unique gifts that he gave to each of them.

Gratitude for what is in our hearts for a deceased loved one can also be high-octane fuel for compassion. It's what often brings fractured families together in their grief — strengthening family bonds. Ironically, it's usually only when a family member dies that relatives put aside their petty differences and gather at the funeral to mourn their shared loss. Funny, how it's often only in death that we come to appreciate life, instead of opening up to the love of those who are still on this earth.

Grief can also be a catalyst for positive action and change. I'm sure that you know of someone who launched a support group or fundraiser after losing a loved one. The bereaved are often motivated to keep the spirit of their loved one alive, to ensure their death wasn't in vain. This action has tremendous healing power, especially for grieving parents. In fact, some of the best social justice movements and non-profits like Mothers Against Drunk Driving (MADD) or Jack.org, a Canadian youth mental health initiative, were born out of the untimely death of a child. Such a profound loss can result in immeasurable gain.

For many of us, our first experience with death will be the loss of a beloved family pet. When your pet dies, something inside you profoundly shifts. No amount of anticipatory grieving can prepare you for the empty heartache.

The loss of a pet becomes an opportunity to teach children the concepts of mortality and impermanence — a dress rehearsal for how to process loss in future.

Death is also a catalyst for authentic, caring conversations that build positive coping skills to deal with the adversity that will inevitably come our way as we progress further into this life. Children can learn helpful ways to say goodbye and internalize that it's okay to feel difficult emotions like grief. After all, death is a natural part of life. Even when life seems dark, you can move through the darkness and experience the bright joy of having a new pet.

My first heart-wrenching grief experience — the loss of my father in my early twenties — was a great personal teacher. Little did I know that the transformational power of grief would surprise me years later when I gave birth to my daughter. At long last, the final few lines of the poem that I'd written before my dad died rang true: *"And one day, dear Dad, when I have my own daughter, I'll teach her the things you would have taught her — for the lessons you shared are always with me. When I look in your eyes, my reflection I see. If this one wish God allows me to behold, it'll be worth much more than a lifetime of gold."*

I take comfort in knowing I've actualized the best of my father's parenting style so my children can know him through me. And I often smile when I see a trait or mannerism of my father's revealing itself in my son or daughter. I now see this relevation is the legacy — the gift in loss — that's always there for me to unwrap.

GETTING GOOD AT GRIEF

"Grief is like a long valley, a winding valley where any bend may reveal a totally new landscape."
— C.S. Lewis

When I lost my dad, the grief section of the bookstore didn't exist. I had no idea how to soothe or heal myself in a healthy way. Instead, I was encouraged to numb my pain — partying, drinking more, throwing myself into my work — to try to forget about my loss. Not only does numbing the pain not work, but it also keeps you suspended in time in a painful place since you're not allowing yourself to move through your grief.

Of course, grief doesn't progress in neat stages that you can tick off, especially if you're doing everything to avoid it. It's helpful to know the possible stages of grief: denial, anger, bargaining, depression and acceptance, first detailed in *On Death and Dying*, the ground-breaking 1969 book by psychiatrist Elisabeth Kübler-Ross.[51] Even though not everyone experiences these stages, let alone in a linear or predictable manner, they can help you understand the major emotional arcs associated with grief. Suffice it to say, grief isn't something you just "get over" as society would like us to believe. Rather, you learn to grow around your grief, walk with it, knowing a wave may return at any time.

I'm sure you've experienced these waves of grief. Maybe you're out in that ocean right now. You feel pulled back in and out of emotional upheaval, like a strong tide. For most of us, the waves last for several months of sorrow, numbness, guilt, or anger, then gradually ease toward acceptance. After six months, more than half of all grievers can move past this acute stage. Yes, there is light and there's some sense of relief. Life still isn't easy, but you can smile again, enjoy a funny memory and consider moving forward without your loved one.

If you're still struggling in your grief a year, or more, after a death, that's okay too. Certain factors can make the grieving process more difficult for some people. These factors include: the circumstances of the death (sudden), closeness of the relationship, your age, past experience with death and the multiplicity of losses/trauma experienced in close proximity. So, if a death is sudden or you had a complicated relationship with the deceased — such as unfinished business — it can be exceptionally difficult to heal.

Let's say the last time you saw your brother, you had a big fight. If he died in a car accident the next day, you wouldn't have had the chance to reconcile or make peace. That unresolved conflict would make it harder for you to come to terms with your grief. The same goes for sudden death — like a plane crash — where there's no opportunity to see the body, say goodbye, make an apology or profess love.

Perhaps the best way to navigate grief is a "one day at a time" approach, only concerning yourself with wherever you are on the roadmap today. Know that one of the most compassionate things that you can do is to allow your grief to unfold. Ask for help from a professional — grief therapist, physician, clergy — if you feel stuck or detoured.

Although your grief experience is uniquely, intimately yours, it often takes a village — a supportive community of family and friends — to help you navigate a clear path. There's always a village of grievers just like you who have suffered a similar loss. Grievers who just might help you uncover the lessons in your own loss, whether you've lost a father, like I did, or a colleague like Frank, your loss is valid and worthy of support.

For now, please be patient and gentle with yourself if you've experienced a recent loss. You're exactly where you need to be. If that's on the couch with a tub of ice cream today, that's okay. I'm right there with you. You never know, you might find a nugget of learning at the bottom of that container, or at least a large chunk of chocolate brownie. Either way, you'll get a good endorphin hit!

With time, you'll learn how to self-soothe and self-heal with the coping strategies that you'll be adding to your toolkit. Start with the strategies listed below that might be as simple as getting a good night's sleep or sharing a good belly laugh with a friend. These strategies are critical mental health tools and good grief resiliency skills that you'll want to access repeatedly.

Rest assured, the darkness will lighten. It won't always be the first thing that you think about when you wake up and the last thought that you have before wrestling your way back to sleep.

GIFT BOX RESILIENCY TOOLS

Below are my top five self-soothing techniques that I encourage you to implement for resilient grieving:

1. **GROUNDING** — At Checkpoint 5, you had the opportunity to practise grounding yourself in your five senses and focusing your attention on your breath. This exercise will also help you to self-soothe by calming your nervous system when you feel overwhelmed by waves of grief.

2. **CIGAR BREATHING** — Pout your lips then breathe deeply in and out through your mouth (count five seconds for both the in and out breath) for at least three minutes. This technique activates the vagus nerve that has the effect of

calming your nervous system, and dissipating fear, anxiety and panic.

3. **SELF-CUDDLE** — Give yourself a butterfly hug by placing the palm of your right hand on your left armpit and the palm of your left hand on your right armpit. Relax your shoulders and squeeze tightly. Feel the warmth of your body through the palms of your hands. Breathe. Hold this position for five seconds while tapping your thumbs lightly on your collar bones, then release. This exercise lowers your heart rate and elevates feelings of safety whenever you're experiencing waves of sadness, abandonment or anxiety.

4. **RITUALS** — Find small, healing ways to keep the spirit of your loved one alive and ease your grief journey. For example, wear their favourite sweater, eat their favourite seasonal foods or plant flowers they liked. In his book, *How We Grieve: Relearning the World*, Dr. Thomas Attig suggests, "Continue to have what you have lost, that is, a continuing, albeit transformed, love for the deceased."[52] You never have to completely sever your connection with your loved one.

5. **GRATITUDE** — Look for good in the world every single day. We learned at Checkpoint 3,

> gratitude fosters well-being. So, taking time every day to write down in a dedicated gratitude journal anything good that remains in your life. Ask yourself, "What am I grateful for today?" Then smile, even if it's forced, for at least thirty seconds. Your body will start to register this real or fake smile as genuine happiness and naturally release healing endorphins.

One of the best lessons that I've learned in grief is that you can still say goodbye to a deceased loved one, long after their death. Aside from the therapeutic benefit of this closure, there are often learning nuggets in the legacy that you can uncover through this process.

I was finally able to do grief therapy several years after my father's passing. With the help of a gifted grief therapist, I worked through years of unresolved grief and unfinished business. Using a Gestalt technique known as the "empty chair monologue," I imagined my dad sitting in a chair across from me, having one final conversation. I did the same at the gravesite of one of my closest friends who died of AIDS. This cathartic process of saying goodbye actualized much-needed closure. The "empty chair" is a therapy technique that I've since employed with hundreds of clients to help melt away years of unresolved grief, anger, guilt, shame and non-acceptance.

🎁 GIFT BOX RESILIENCY TOOLS

Here's how you could do the "empty chair" exercise yourself or with the help of a therapist. Please know it can bring up painful memories that may require professional support. Yet, the result may surprise you with insights about your relationship, what mattered most and what you will cherish moving forward — the unexpected gifts.

- Write a letter to your deceased loved one detailing everything you ever wanted to tell them or say to them before their death. Describe the ways they've influenced your life.

- Read the letter aloud to them with their photo in an empty chair across from you.

- Alternatively, you can go to the gravesite where your loved one is buried, or where their ashes may be, and read the letter aloud to them.

- Journal your feelings and thoughts upon completion of this exercise. Please reach out for support if you're feeling overwhelmed.

COMPLICATED GRIEF (SUICIDE, MISCARRIAGE AND PET LOSS)

"Sorrow is less of a checklist, more like water. It's fluid, it has no set shape, never disappears, never ends. It doesn't go away. It just changes. It changes us."
— Mira Ptacin

I took the first plane that I could. I'd been living in the Arctic when I received the call that one of my dearest friends, Michael, had lost his battle with HIV-AIDS. He only had days to live. As the airport taxi approached Toronto General Hospital, a wave of despair washed over me. Somehow, intuitively, I knew that I hadn't made it in time. Michael passed away while I was en route. I arrived an hour too late to say goodbye.

He was a sparkly, feisty, hundred-watt-lightbulb type of friend. The kind of friend who sits with a baseball bat by your door all night after your condo has been robbed. The friend who shops with you for those one-of-a kind shoes, dances with you until sunrise and who helps you whip up a chocolate souffle at the last minute. Simply irreplaceable.

Michael was from a strict Greek Macedonian family and had hidden his sexual orientation from them for all his adult life. After his death, Michael's family whisked his body back to his childhood hometown where only close family were invited to attend a closed memorial service. They didn't consider the bereavement needs of his partner and many beloved friends. His family refused to acknowledge that he had died of AIDS, choosing instead to say he had died of cancer.

When we're excluded from the opportunity to say goodbye or to mourn, we often experience feelings of helplessness, frustration and disempowerment. The kind of circumstances that create what's known as "disenfranchised grief" — an unacknowledged mourner (e.g., LGBTQI+ partner of someone who was not out), a stigmatized death like suicide/drug overdose, or a death considered less important or tragic (e.g., loss of a pet).

My work in trauma intervention means that I'm often asked to help employees learn what to say or not to say to be helpful, especially regarding topics that may still be considered taboo, such as suicide, miscarriage, stillborn birth, addictions, Alzheimer's, severe mental illness, or the death of someone who's imprisoned or convicted of a crime. Other non-death losses that cause harmful, long-lasting distress include loss of mobility/health, your home and possessions, your independence, an unsuccessful adoption or fertility treatment.

Disenfranchised grief is particularly difficult to overcome without supportive family, friends, or community. That's why we need to connect on a human scale with anyone and everyone who may be suffering regardless of the circumstances or situation. Loving kindness and compassion for yourself and all beings is a key ingredient for good grief. Compassion is usually needed the most by those who we think don't deserve it. The practice of being non-judgmental is perhaps the best way to free yourself and all grievers from the prison of silent tears and self-stigma. This practice will pave the way for all future mourners to cope better and uncover the unexpected gift in their grief.

So, if you'd like more support for disenfranchised losses, namely, death by suicide, miscarriage, or loss of a pet, please turn to the Good Grief Parking Lot found in the downloadable resources kit at www.catherineclarkconnects.com. You'll be able to read more vulnerable stories and practise Coffee with Catherine tools to help support you in these stigmatized grief situations.

Now that we've navigated our way through this arduous journey called grief, let's gas up and get back on the resiliency roadway. At the next exit, we will look at how to build a solid network of caring connections with others and, most importantly, a loving relationship with ourselves. This solid network will not only support us through times of great loss but also propel us to experience great joy.

CHECKPOINT 9

Deconstructing Disconnections – Cultivating Connections

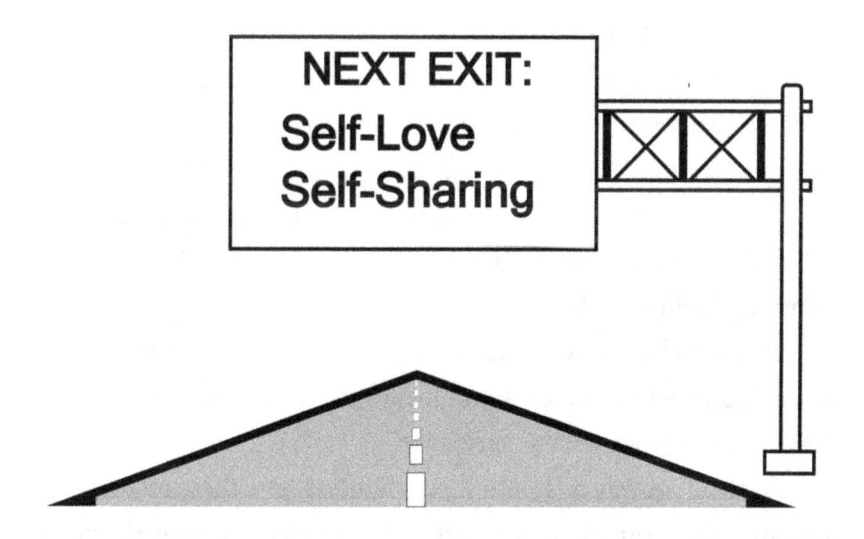

NEXT EXIT:
Self-Love
Self-Sharing

"We humans are social beings. We come into the world as the result of others' actions. We survive here in dependence on others. Whether we like it or not, there is hardly a moment of our lives when we do not benefit from others' activities. For this reason it is hardly surprising that most of our happiness arises in the context of our relationships with others."
— *The Dalai Lama XIV*

As social beings, we are all hardwired for human connection and belonging. Brené Brown defines this social state as, "The energy that exists between people when they feel seen, heard and valued; when they can give and receive without judgement; and when they derive sustenance and strength from a relationship."[32] Our neurons, hormones and genetics drive us toward connection — interdependence over independence.

I believe the most crucial ingredient for mental health resiliency is, first and foremost, to love yourself and then have the unwavering belief that you are loved unconditionally. And you've certainly been gathering tools to help with that.

At Checkpoint 8, we described the grief we experience when someone we love dies. In psychological terms, we also experience profound trauma when a close friendship or romantic relationship ends — one of our darkest packages. In fact, the brain chemistry experienced is the same as if this person had died. A breakup also brings up feelings of being pushed away and rejected into full view for everyone else to see. It becomes a public heartbreak where you feel judged — like there's something wrong with you — severed, disconnected from your secure base.

At this highway exit, let's shed a light on how these relationship disconnections can be opportunities for enormous personal growth — dark gifts. Yes, we're on the home stretch — cruising home to you. We'll talk briefly about what breeds disconnection — powerlessness and self-abandonment. No big surprises here. Then we'll learn the foundation needed for healthy caring connections, namely self-love. You can finally get rid of anything else in your trunk that weighs you down and no longer serves you. After all, only strong, nurturing relationships are needed in your vehicle moving forward. That's better for you and better for your gas mileage, too.

HUMAN CONNECTION DEFICIT SYNDROME

Human Connection Deficit Syndrome (HCDS) is a term I coined during the Covid-19 pandemic to describe the feeling of profound disconnection, isolation and apathy due to lowered levels of happy chemicals like dopamine, oxytocin and serotonin that are released via human touch and social interaction. At our core, we have a biological craving for human connection. When the pandemic dragged on, I thought we needed a way to describe this deep disconnectedness.

In his 2011 TED Talk, Dr. Paul Zak, a renowned neuroscientist, prescribed at least eight hugs per day to feel happier and more connected, to help our brains experience trust, and to encourage prosocial behaviours such as generosity, compassion and forgiveness — all critical elements of the Mental Health Resiliency Roadmap.

Let's face it, loneliness is becoming a huge stressor in all of our lives. It's exacerbated if we can't physically be with other human beings, or we can't find the time to forge caring relationships. After the 2020 pandemic hit, medical researchers began predicting that this dark package — called loneliness — will be the next biggest public health epidemic of our time. However, mental health advocates like myself are optimistic that because of Covid-19, loneliness will finally be given the mainstream recognition it deserves — possibly paving the way for a more socially connected future and much needed mental health resources.

Many of us pretend to be happy. When in reality, we feel very, very alone. And HCDS, like loneliness, is a great masquerader.

HCDS is not necessarily someone sitting alone in their apartment by themselves. It can look like irritability, depression, withdrawal, lack of focus, impulsivity, sleep disturbance, obesity and addiction. We're not just observing this syndrome in our families and co-workers today. Now teachers are also seeing these mental health challenges in elementary-school-aged children.

All told, we absolutely require human connection — supportive relationships — to not only help us thrive but also to keep us alive. In my suicide hotline experience, what keeps someone on the phone is to get them talking about one person (even their dog) who would really miss them — someone who cares if they live or die. The Centers for Disease Control and Prevention (CDC) found that "connectedness" is also one of the most important mitigating factors in suicide prevention.

The CDC describes connectedness as, "The degree to which a person or group is socially close, interrelated, or shares resources with one another." So, shopping for groceries for a neighbour, sharing home renovation tools or a community garden are all easy ways to alleviate loneliness. Or something as simple as grabbing a weekly cup of coffee or going for a walk with a friend, could mitigate HCDS and possibly save a life — yours included.

Not to geek out on research, but a 2015 meta-analysis of studies on loneliness determined that living with loneliness increases our odds of dying prematurely.[53] Crazy to believe, but true. Feeling lonely doesn't mean there's something wrong with you. It's usually caused by heartbreak, personal loss or self-isolation. We can combat mounting loneliness by identifying and nurturing quality, caring relationships. That may even be having a dog or cat to cuddle every day because a human-animal bond can be a stronger connection for some people than a human-human bond.

So, here's the thing: we can start to lessen HCDS when we take better care of our existing friendship networks and work team connections now. Even nurturing long-distance bonds online can help us weather the inevitable ups and downs, tragedies and transitions of life. I have heard it said that we get by with the help of our friends.

So, let's stop at the gift shop now and pick up some tools to help us combat HCDS and this dark package called loneliness.

🎁 GIFT BOX RESILIENCY TOOLS

Some creative ways to address Human Connection Deficit Syndrome (HCDS) and improve our mental health include:

1. Reach out regularly to someone you love, especially if you suspect they are struggling too, and say, "Even if we cannot physically be together, I see you, I hear you, I deeply value you and I love you." Send this message in a text, voice memo or handwrite it in a card and mail it. See if your mood improves with just this one action.

2. Ask one person in your life to be your confidant and accountability buddy. This person could be a family member, friend, co-worker, someone from an online support group or a therapist — someone you trust implicitly.

3. If you live alone, find someone you can share a meal with, or a walk, once a week. together.

4. Set up a regular weekly (or more frequent) check-in time or chat time via Zoom with your buddy. Send regular voice memos back and forth so you can hear voice inflection and share a laugh (endorphins).

5. Purchase a weighted blanket to lay across your chest and shoulders to mimic a hug. This blanket can help you feel much calmer and nurtured.

6. Pet an animal like a dog or cat to lower anxiety and release oxytocin – another good reason to be a pet parent or visit the doggy park.

7. Find an online group that regularly meets and plays a game, like trivia night, or shares funny stories/comedy with one another.

8. Take a walk in nature and hug a tree. Feel the rocky mountain high or calming effect of being near water. Nature can make you feel more connected to the earth, regulate blood pressure, reduce stress and boost mental health.

9. Observe human touch in others. Whether in real life, or virtually, observing touch can give you many of the same benefits as actually feeling touch.

10. Volunteer to help at a homeless shelter, do the grocery shopping for an elderly neighbour, offer to take your neighbour's kids to the park or doggy sit. Research has shown that happy hormones and brain activity increase when volunteering. Connecting with like-minded individuals through volunteering can also reduce feelings of loneliness and create a kindness chain.

RELATIONSHIP DISCONNECTIONS — OUT OF THE DARK

*"When someone shows you who they are,
believe them the first time."*
— Maya Angelou

Thinking back to some of the client stories we've talked about so far on this road trip, you may recognize the tactics of a deeply disconnected relationship. Perhaps you see yourself or your friends in a very toxic partnership.

What's interesting to me is how we can live most of our lives trying to be in the type of relationship or social group that makes us look like we "belong" or we've "made it" on the outside. Yet, we have no "inner-belonging" — it's like we're complete strangers in our own house. We feel painfully disconnected from ourselves, who we are, what we're passionate about and what matters most to us. It's feeling invisible — a gnawing loneliness — whether you're in a room full of people or sleeping next to a partner that you've been married to for twenty years.

This feeling of deep disconnection is further exacerbated when we've been abandoned by a partner or can't find a way out of a soul-crushing relationship. Throughout this book, I have mentioned abusive relationships — a type of deep disconnection. At this exit, I want to focus on ways for you to reconnect with yourself and start to rock your life after leaving an abusive relationship. So, if you've already suffered at the hands of an abusive partner, please know you can heal. There is light in this dark package, and a better understanding of the abuse cycle may aid in your recovery process. It might help to persuade you that you are a victim and not merely a participant in the whole episode.

As we know, leaving any relationship can be excruciatingly difficult — even more so if it's an abusive relationship. Coined by Dr. Lenore E. Walker in the late 1970s, the "cycle of abuse" describes the tension-building, acting-out, reconciliation/honeymoon and calm cycling throughout the majority of abusive relationships. Narcissistic abuse is one of the most insidious forms of domestic violence, as abusers are typically charming, attractive and able to morph into whatever personality is needed for them to get what they want. The only way to regain your sense of self is to fully disconnect from a narcissist and break the destructive cycle.[54]

I have provided you with some additional information in the downloadable resources kit at www.catherineclarkconnects.com, which will help you recognize the narcissistic abuse cycle and learn the strategies needed to take a stand and leave. There are professional supports available at each and every step of the way. Once you have this guidance, you can completely reinvest in yourself.

Believe me, I'm still learning and growing alongside you. This is a lifelong learning highway of refuelling and course correcting.

MOVING FORWARD — UNWRAPPING THE DARK GIFT

"Someone I loved once gave me a box full of darkness.
It took me years to understand that this too, was a gift."
— Mary Oliver, *The Uses of Sorrow*

You'll know you're healing from a toxic relationship when you feel safe and so much lighter — you can genuinely smile and reconnect with beautiful YOU again.

So, yes, things do get better. If you're able to fully immerse yourself in this dark box, feel the pain, face your demons and uncover your programming that says, "You need to give up your voice to be loved," and you just might find your authentic self.

Finding your authentic self likely won't happen overnight. Recovery and healing look different for everyone. It's normal to feel traumatized and confused for a period afterwards, which could be months or even years. Just know that being in a toxic relationship can feel like being in a constant state of "fight, flight or freeze," where your sympathetic nervous system is constantly firing and working overtime. Once you have some distance from an abusive relationship, your parasympathetic nervous system starts to kick in. This system creates a calming "rest and digest" response — the soil needed to plant seeds of self-love again; a beautiful garden of yellow roses. So, how will you grow?

You'll have a whole new confident mindset.
One of the best gifts to emerge from leaving a toxic relationship is that you get to the other side with a fuller, stronger, version of yourself. Not to mention feeling like a bad-ass, take-no-prisoners boss.

You're physically healthier.
You may be pleasantly surprised, and relieved, that chronic physical conditions like headaches, joint pain and gastrointestinal issues start to resolve once your body feels safe again. I had people regularly say to me, "You seem so much more relaxed since you left that abusive relationship, Catherine." And now I understand why. What a relief to be out of the eye of the storm!

You learn that boundaries are healthy.
When you're finally finished being a doormat, you quickly learn that clear parameters and nailed-down boundaries are your golden rules. You can say, "hell no" and mean it. And if someone tries to cross your line or doesn't respect you, then you have no problem showing them the door.

You know how to spot and deal with narcissists.
You'll have a nailed-down strategy for dealing with people who have high narcissistic traits. Yes, they usually have a "preferred type" they target and you're probably the "empath" who fits the bill. I sure know I am! So, look around and apply similar boundaries to all those relationships in your life. You might even want to consider weeding people out of your garden completely. Start by revisiting some of the boundary-setting techniques we picked up at Checkpoint 6.

You learn communication strategies to deal with toxic people.
Using a communication technique known as the "Grey Rock" method might help keep you disengaged. The trick is to think of yourself as emotionally detached like a non-responsive, boring, grey rock. My therapist also introduced me to the visual of acting

like a stealthy, Bombay cat, confidently swaggering across the top of a fence — completely unbothered by the guard dog below. This response takes away what an abuser needs and craves the most — attention and power.

You channel your pain for good.
Once you can move beyond your pain, you may want to help others who have been harmed in toxic relationships or are trying to leave. You now have the gift of hindsight. You recognize the signs of an abusive relationship and can help others do the same. This recognition often motivates you to serve your highest good, which we will explore at our last Checkpoint 11.

Please know that it's normal for your journey back to yourself to take many directions, twists and turns. You've taken a big step on this road trip by even acknowledging and making peace with relationship disconnections.

So, now, let's get to the good stuff — falling in love with YOU. We'll start by looking at an example of a client who moved from disconnection to finding a beautiful new connection with herself.

GETTING TO SELF-LOVE

> *"What a lovely surprise to finally discover
> how unlonely being alone can be."*
> — Ellen Burstyn

Nadine, a well-manicured woman in her mid-forties, came to see me at a point when she had no other choice than to throw out her previous life roadmap, graduate from hurtful patterns and get on a whole new road trip.

"I'm all alone. I feel unlovable." These words spilled out of Nadine's mouth as she allowed herself to experience the full weight of her broken marriage. Two weeks earlier her husband of seventeen years had shocked her with the news that he was leaving her for another woman. Nadine could not even entertain the thought of her life as a single woman again. So much of her self-worth had been tied to her husband's financial success, his reputation in the community and her seemingly perfect, curated world. As the saying goes, Nadine had put all her eggs in one basket — a romantic relationship with her partner. She had focused all her energy on her husband while her career had taken a complete backseat. So much so that his world became her entire world. The obvious downside of that occurs when you lose your partner, you feel as though you've lost everything, especially your self-esteem.

Nadine sought counselling at just the right time. With the help of cognitive behavioural therapy, she was able to channel her intense anger and target her negative self-talk to develop a whole new self-concept. So, Nadine did not stay stuck for long in the psychological neutral stage of transition. She collected up the parts of herself that she had disowned in her marriage. Little by little, her story became one of self-love. She was ready to begin anew by investing energy into cultivating her own self-worth. Nadine faced her fears, created new opportunities for growth and completely relaunched her own career.

The good news is that you can write a new love story at any age. And if your dark package is a relationship breakdown, starting today, you can develop a caring connection with yourself. You can celebrate being self-partnered, an alternative for the word single. It was popularized by actress Emma Watson in a November 2019 interview with British Vogue. In that interview, Watson called out how society often judges women who are single, as if something is wrong with them for not finding or wanting a partner. It speaks volumes that, at only thirty years of age, Watson felt the weight of societal pressure to marry and have a home, two children and a stable career. In many cultures, a woman is only considered fully thriving when she has found someone who loves her and wants to marry her — "put a ring on it."

Yup, that's the bandwagon I hopped on many years ago, too. Now, I'm transitioning again from being married for twenty-three years to being a self-partnered, empty-nester — seemingly overnight. So, I can hear post-traumatic growth knocking at my door again.

When my marriage ended, I promised myself that I would learn to be with just "me." Learn how to enjoy my alone time again — which is completely different from being lonely. Learn to have dates with myself. Learn to live in a space full of gratitude for every new day and build my mental health resilience with a solid foundation of self-love.

"You, yourself, as much as anybody in the entire universe, deserve your love and affection."
— Buddha

How do we learn to love?

Perhaps you developed your concept of love from a Hollywood, happily ever after, "you complete me" script too? Or maybe the iconic Tiffany box declaration of love is the tape that plays in your subconscious. Every one of us has a very different definition and experience of love. Understanding your concept of love is like chiselling away at a sculpture to uncover the precise actions that you associate with this word. As a young child, you sponged up a range of behaviours that you internalized as your love language by watching your parents or caregivers. In my case, I had two parents who were very affectionate towards one another, worked well together as partners and seemed to epitomize a loving partnership.

But what I also internalized was codependency.

My Mom was completely reliant on my Dad for so many of her basic needs, and when my dad was happy, her self-esteem soared. She doted on everyone — in typical fifties housewife fashion — wanting only what was best for her family. She was the role model of self-sacrificing behaviour, while often ignoring her own needs completely.

It wasn't her fault. This behaviour was the social conditioning she passed along that she'd been taught, and so the social conditioning continues when we don't change the script.

This behaviour also meant that people-pleasing, obsessing about your children's behavioural outcomes and enforcing rules that prevent open expression of differences were deeply imprinted, too. While looking for love in places outside yourself is second nature, you'll never feel fulfilled if you can't love yourself first from the inside out.

I've come to realize that this template for loving behaviour has been in the background all my life. Although my idea of love hasn't necessarily changed, per se, my sense of self-love has certainly evolved. Looking in the mirror, I'm not at all the same person I was when I married for the first time at age twenty-seven. I look at pictures of myself back then and say, "Wow, I don't even know who that person is anymore." I'm betting you feel the same way too.

Looking back, I'm reminded of how much I've grown inside as a spiritual being. How much I've grown to love and appreciate the core, vulnerable, inner ME. How I've grown to know my deepest fears and desires. How I've grown to have such deep respect for myself. At this checkpoint, you can start to embody self-love in your own way too.

Self-love first and foremost means practising self-acceptance, self-compassion and self-forgiveness — tools that we already put in our resiliency toolkit at Checkpoint 2.

When you accept yourself in this very moment — with droopy eyelids and bad hair — you're practising self-love. This is hard to do if you're magnified on a large Zoom screen every day. And yes, it means working on accepting your weaknesses without having to explain away all the shortcomings. I look forward to the day when we can all stop apologizing for something — a wrinkled shirt, smudged mascara, or a lapse in memory. The truth is, when you can forgive yourself and hold yourself in high esteem, you're more likely to continue to choose things that nurture self-love and help you thrive.

Self-love also means accepting your emotions for what they are and putting your physical, emotional and mental well-being first — as we learned to do at Checkpoint 1. It's also being more compassionate toward both ourselves and others as human beings who are struggling to find meaning and purpose in our lives. Remembering we all suffer — we all feel "lesser than" at some point. Compassion is at the core of how we evolve to a more affirming place of self-fulfillment. We'll be digging deeper into this concept at the last checkpoint — Checkpoint 11.

I'm so honoured that you're still with me on this roller-coaster ride of a resiliency road trip. Starting today, you can nurture your relationship with amazing YOU! Baby steps are all that's required here. If you're in a place where it's really hard to love yourself right now, that's okay. Self-love is a muscle that you build up slowly. It's not a quantum leap but a consistent "micro-moments" practice.

Let's stop at the coffee shop now to talk about the small ways we can make it easier to love ourselves. Not just when we succeed and things go as planned, but also when we mess up and our lives completely fall apart.

☕ COFFEE WITH CATHERINE

We can tap into self-love by reflecting on what it looks and feels like to be unconditionally loved with these coaching prompts:

1. Bring to mind a specific person or memory where you felt unconditionally loved. For some of us, this may be a relationship with a companion animal. How would this person or creature act toward you if they knew that you were struggling? What would they be saying or doing to demonstrate their love? How would they communicate admiration, compassion and acceptance toward you?

2. Think about how you can practise being that same person for yourself, a true friend. Bring to mind a time when you encouraged yourself and really admired what you had accomplished. As you go throughout your day, pause and find moments where you can admire and encourage yourself. Then sit with this feeling, letting it sink into your body. Breathe. Smile. The more you do this, the more you deliberately reprogram your brain to experience the feeling of being loving and on your own side.
3. Have you been comparing yourself to others? Comparison is a self-love killer. Instead of measuring your flaws against someone else's strengths, you can nourish your own unique gifts and successes. Make a realistic list of the qualities that other people cherish, value, promote and love about you. Ask a friend to help you brainstorm.
4. What would your best friend say are your most fascinating, unique qualities? Now say each one out loud to me or to yourself in the mirror. "I am _____ and _____." Now say, "I love you (your name), unconditionally."
5. Accept the parts of yourself that you simply cannot love yet. You don't need to love everything about yourself to develop self-love; all you need is acceptance.

6. Build a path to self-love by taking baby steps — small daily actions — that stir joy, create excitement and make you feel like you're really taking care of yourself.
7. Next time something happens that makes you want to get down on yourself, challenge yourself to accept what is. So, instead of even aiming to love those parts of yourself, where your mind goes, "Are you kidding me?" simply focus on accepting them. Instead, you could say, "I accept all of me unconditionally just as I am."
8. You could tell yourself something along the lines of, "It's okay, I can be unhappy with some parts of myself in this situation. It's not the end of the world."
9. Practise loving with the same wholeheartedness and sympathetic concern you'd have for a friend.
10. Realize that by caring for yourself, your actions have a positive ripple effect on everyone else around you. Make a list of who might be positively affected by greater self-love (e.g., your daughter, friend, co-worker, etc.).

GIFT BOX RESILIENCY TOOLS

Top ten tools to quickly amp up your self-love and feel great about yourself again:

1. Tell yourself that your value doesn't lie in your appearance.
2. Prioritize your self-care and set healthy boundaries.
3. Say "yes" to new life experiences, both joyful and painful.
4. Let go of toxic people.
5. Make mistakes with curiosity — let go of self-judgement.
6. Stop comparing yourself to others or listening to their opinions instead of tuning into your own needs.
7. Trust yourself to make good decisions that are best for you.
8. Speak your mind and speak up for what you deserve.
9. Forgive yourself and stop apologizing.
10. Channel your inner rock star — dance, dance, dance!

SELF-LOVE IS THE NEW SEXY

Being self-partnered and growing in self-love has been one of the best gifts to come from my recent separation. To be honest, it really is the new sexy. It might not happen overnight, but with "mirror work" and consistent positive self-talk, the depth of love that you have for yourself just might surprise you one day. At least that's how it happened for me.

In the summer of 2021, I took a break from writing to clear my head and walk along Lake Ontario. The Great Lakes are instant, awe-inspiring, spiritual grounders. As I ambled along the waterfront in what was then my new neighbourhood — taking in all the sensations — I felt a sudden surge of endorphins. It was that tingly sort of first day, romantic love feeling pulsating from my heart center. My lungs started to expand with gratitude as I breathed in the clean lake air. My soul felt so much lighter. My spirit was speaking to me with each carefree step that I took. It was a faint voice at first, getting closer, louder and then fully joy-struck. "What the heck? I'm actually feeling happy and very, very grateful." I felt giddy with love!

I was falling in love with ME!

For the first time, maybe ever, I closed my eyes and took a deep breath from my whole heart and felt waves of renewing self-love. I started to spontaneously recite out loud the loving kindness meditation that I had been regularly practising. I said to myself, "I am happy, I am healthy, I am living with greater ease and I am truly at peace." I stood there with my eyes wide open, consciously observing myself — observing this moment. I was connecting to my innermost being, my wants and needs, a deep trust in the universe — a belief in all the infinite possibilities that lie ahead. I had been gifted heart wrenching darkness so my own heart could discover an inner light.

I bravely let go of any "lesser than" or "single again" judgement and further boosted my mood with a happy little lakeshore dance. I quoted motivational speaker, Lisa Nichols' famous line, "What other people think of me is none of my business." I could finally speak from a place of healed scars instead of open wounds. I let out a giant "YES!" as I stood basking in the heavenly view, feeling love from my crown chakra to my toes. It was a powerful "knowing" — my biggest step forward in my own healing journey.

I believe the moment that you realize you have fallen in love with yourself — in love with life — you will see all other areas of your life fall into place as well. Your career or business will start thriving, other people around you will start loving you more, the world will look more beautiful and the sun will shine brighter.

Conscious self-love clears the way to fully experience all the love in the world — inside and out — to self-share in an adaptive, affirming way. So, let's dig into self-sharing and all the healthy ways that we can foster loving relationships with others. Let's mindfully choose the kind of friendships and caring connections that support good mental health and endless joy. Amen to that!

CULTIVATING LOVING FRIENDSHIPS

> *"Friends are the family you choose."*
> — Jess C. Scott

> *"A true friend knows your weaknesses but shows you your strengths; feels your fears but fortifies your faith; sees your anxieties but frees your spirit; recognizes your disabilities but emphasizes your possibilities."*
> — William Arthur Ward

Reaching out to friends for support, advice and encouragement is vital to overcoming adversity. Resilience is not about heroically toughing it out alone. Having a strong network of supportive family and friends just might save your life. I'm only here today because my oldest and dearest friend, Laurie, literally thwarted my suicide plan.

Cultivating loving connections requires the capacity to self-share — to risk being vulnerable enough to share your innermost world with others. This kind of sharing means being open, authentic and trusting. It also demands a willingness to create an authentic, safe space for sharing. Holding space can be very challenging for people in this increasingly digital age. It takes time, courage and effort to openly share yourself — your past mistakes, embarrassments and even your proudest moments — with another person.

Sharing yourself with others (self-share) is like building up a "trust bank account."

Cultivating friendship requires regular deposits to your trust bank account. The initial investment in your friendship takes a lot of effort, but thereafter it compounds exponentially to make you very wealthy in the years to come. And once a friendship is well-established, you still must keep making regular deposits, just not as frequently.

Let's look at how one of my clients found a way to build a trust bank account and weather the loneliness of the Covid-19 pandemic with a newfound friendship.

Omar, a twenty-nine-year-old stockbroker— whom I supported telephonically during the Covid-19 lockdown — mitigated loneliness and forged new relationships by finding a "bubble buddy." This buddy is a person or a family you choose to have regular contact with either in your own apartment building/neighbourhood or in your wider friendship network. During a lockdown it was a safe way to share meals, resources and fellowship with brand new or existing friends.

Omar became bubble buddies with a neighbourhood couple in his highrise apartment building who had a small baby. He regularly shared groceries, cooking and babysitting so that his new friends could enjoy a walk together and much-needed couple time. Omar's dark gift was discovering just how much he loved babies and his future desire to find a partner who shared his newfound love for children. He described this discovery as a complete departure from the previous attitude that he held about having children. Omar also rediscovered his joy of playing board games and taking the time to enjoy a home cooked meal with friends who made him laugh. He realized the deep capacity he had for nurturing close, trusting relationships. He vowed to make these types of relationships his new priority.

Omar's positive experience with cultivating a caring connection during such a difficult time reminds me of a saying in Okinawa, the sub-tropical Japanese islands, that goes something like this:

"Live far enough away from your family so you're not running into them every day, but close enough to take them a warm bowl of soup on foot."

Perhaps the Okinawans have discovered the secret to mental health resiliency. They have large families and strong social support networks. Their communities are really close-knit and everybody knows everybody. They have social gatherings in groups known as "moai." They regularly chat about common interests, drink green tea and share meals. That's right up my alley. According to Dr. Bradley J. Willcox, who co-authored *The Okinawa Way*, keeping close connections and socializing has been found to be one of the key contributors to why these island inhabitants have the highest concentrations of centenarians in the world.[55]

So, if you live in a large city, you're probably shaking your head right now. But, look at the great experience Omar had by stepping out of his comfort zone and going against his typical "keep to yourself" apartment culture. There are so many ways to build community — a tiny tribe within smaller neighbourhoods of a larger centre — like a community garden, little league baseball or art in the park. Co-operative housing complexes — where every person contributes to the beautification and functioning of the building — offer endless opportunities for connectedness.

Irrespective of where we live, friendships are a critical component of our overall health and wellness. It's worth repeating that having a strong network of supportive family and friends helps enhance our resilience and bolsters our mental health. Friends pass you a flashlight to help you find your way through any dark night. They hold up a three-way mirror that puts your life back in focus when you've lost all perspective.

All you really need in life is just one person who has your back; a person with whom you can be fully, authentically raw, undressed and unapologetically YOU.

Developing this kind of deep relationship is easier said than done. We're all in different places on the caring connections continuum today. Some of us have a really trustworthy friend or a family member who we're confidant will help us out in any situation. You know, the person you can call in the middle of the night to bail you out of jail — no questions asked. If you're just starting to realize this need, that's okay. As you build on your mental health resiliency skills, you'll be better able to identify relationships where you can nurture these trust bank accounts.

I was in my late twenties when I met my moai — Warren, Ron, Randi, Michael and Michele — the "Montreal Gang" of twenty-somethings. Together, we celebrated Thanksgiving, we Octoberfested, skied and hiked the Laurentians, jazzfested, danced and brunched our way through Montreal. Honestly, we were kind of like an episode from the TV show *Friends*. These friends are a blessed collection of souls who have sustained me through all of life's ups and downs — all those bloody dark packages. After my first marriage went up in flames, it was this close-knit collection of friends who single-handedly sorted through my condo possessions, loaded up the truck and moved me into a funky new apartment.

Friends might help you pack or make reservations, but "soulmate friends" are there on moving day and beyond. You know you have salt-of-the earth friends when two of the strongest hoist your washing machine up three flights of stairs. Thanks to Simon, I now realize we need friends with superhuman strength, as well. So, remember to put a couple of weightlifters or mountain climbers on your friendship wish list.

Suffice it to say, awesome friends make the world a better place. They help you feel safe to love yourself, to mature as a human being and to open up to the full experience of life. It takes courage to walk through the fear of emotional intimacy — to be authentically you. But, I can't think of any other risk that will pay you back in dividends more than the risk of being a vulnerable friend.

American psychologist, Dr. Donald P. Oswald, found there are four key maintenance behaviours that sustain your "trust bank account" and deepen close connections: positivity, supportiveness, openness and regular interaction. According to Oswald, friendships that regularly and instinctively apply these forms of friendship maintenance, forge the strongest friendship bonds and have higher emotional intimacy.[56]

In his eye-opening book, *On Being Awesome: A Unified Theory of How Not to Suck*, which I would wholeheartedly recommend you read, Nick Riggle, a philosophy professor, brings this concept to life. Riggle describes people who always try to get you to go to their pity party (sucky people) versus the ones who are at the pivot party (awesome people). According to Riggle, "Being awesome is being good at creating "social openings" — moments of mutual appreciation between people when they break out of their norms and routines by expressing their individuality in a way that gets others to express theirs." [57]

Awesome people surprise a friend with an unexpected gift or talk to a stranger in a line-up. They're not preference dictators or fun squelchers. I have been blessed to have both old and new friends in my life who meet the definition of awesome: they're open-minded, curious, optimistic, reliable, good listeners and somehow make you feel worthy just by being in their presence.

So, let's stop at the gift shop and identify whether or not you have awesome friends. Grab your journal. Once you've written about your awesome friends why not give them a call, send a text or voice memo to let them know you love and appreciate them. A little care goes a very long way on our lifelong road trip.

GIFT BOX RESILIENCY TOOLS

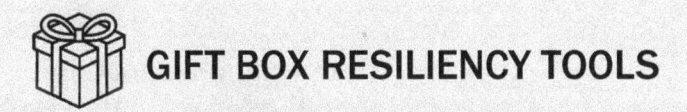

Here are some qualities that I'd like you to consider when choosing an awesome friend with whom to self-share.

If you already have a friend who matches these traits, write their name beside the question. Describe how this person demonstrates these qualities, or how they act in an opposite way. Write down an example of a time when you have also demonstrated these same qualities with your friends.

Does your friend:

1. **Motivate you to pursue your goals or go to the next level?** Are they also committed to their own goals and purpose? This mindset describes my friend Tracy, hands down! She asks me what important project I'm working on and then asks me what small steps I'm taking to achieve a specific goal.

2. **Share similar values?** High level important stuff, like honesty and integrity. Helping others and cultural diversity. Remember, "You're the average of the five people you spend the most time with," as motivational speaker Jim Rohn professes. My Mom is one of my best friends who leads with honesty.

3. **Respect your differences, opinions and preferences?** They remember your food likes and dislikes. My friend Randi is a person who always has café au lait, dark chocolate, Pinot Noir and laughter at the ready.

4. **Make you feel like you can be 100 per cent yourself and honest with them?** You can say "hell no" instead of agreeing with them and saying yes? My friend Denise starts a sentence with, "You can completely reject this suggestion ..." — love that.

5. **Get your quirks, oddities and weird sense of humour and make you laugh so hard that you lose it completely or you pee your pants?** And they're quirky right back — that's right, Michele, this one's for you. As a very introverted artisan, she once paid me the highest compliment by saying, "Being with you, Catherine, is almost as great as being by myself." Go figure.

6. **Check in with you and keep in touch?** Even more frequently when you're socially isolated or down on your luck? My oldest friend, Laurie, has never stopped calling, emailing and writing words of encouragement to me since our earliest university days.

7. **Celebrate your success?** Clap the loudest when you win? As Oscar Wilde said, *"Anybody can sympathize with the sufferings of a friend, but it requires a very fine nature to sympathize with a friend's success."* Honestly, no one makes more noise or pulls out the entire cheerleading, social media team more than Anesh.

8. **Help you course-correct?** Props you up on your worst day? Helps you see things from a new perspective? I'm so blessed to always have my sister, Wendy, by my side — staying up until midnight to read up on divorce law and move logistics.

9. **Stand by you in the tough times, not just the fun times?** You can call them at 2 a.m. Warren owns this category. He's always the first person to get on a plane when your marriage implodes, or you've completely lost it.

10. **Express gratitude, really value your friendship and thank you?** My friend, Becky, reminds me every time we chat how very appreciative she is of our friendship and what I may have said or done that has brightened her world.

Of course, once you can clearly identify the qualities you want and deserve in an awesome friend, you may just be ready to date again — self-share with a friend who becomes an intimate partner. How exiting is that? I'm not suggesting that you rush out and buy up the lingerie department — unless that's part of your own self-love plan. You go girl!

I'll be basking in unwavering self-love and plan to hang out with my "self-stand" buddies for a few more resiliency road trips. Let's spice things up now with a crème brûlée latte and ponder a few intimate relationship questions if you're considering dating again.

☕ COFFEE WITH CATHERINE

Below are my top ten intimate relationship-building questions:

1. How will you know when you're in a loving, flourishing relationship? If you woke up in one tomorrow, what would be the first sign? What would you and your partner say or do?
2. What would a deep emotional, honest, truthful connection with your partner look like? How would your conversations go?
3. Are there any barriers that you're still putting up or wounds you need to heal to allow yourself to be fully loved?
4. What patriarchal values, or toxic role models for intimate relationships, would you need to leave behind so you don't lose yourself or shrink in a partnership?

5. What makes you feel stressed in a relationship?
6. What makes you feel adored in a relationship?
7. What would the unspoken rules or agreements be in your ideal relationship?
8. What are your relationship deal breakers (e.g., smoking, sexually incompatible, not family-oriented, dislikes socializing, etc.)?
9. How would you describe your communication style? Do you avoid hard conversations? How will you bring up and discuss difficult topics and conflicts with your partner so they don't fester?
10. Ten years from now what would a deeply connected, flourishing relationship look like?

Wow, you've just completed some really important work. I learned so much about you in our last coffee chat and I'm excited for the relationships that you'll be building in the near future.

Sometimes life is about being alone and creating a loving relationship with yourself — and sometimes life is about partnering, and socializing with others. Alone and yet together — life presents many juxtapositions. At different points in our lives we have different needs. More than anything, let's acknowledge how hard it can be to not lose yourself in seeking life-enhancing love and support from others. Its a lifetime balancing act. Now that we recognize the critical ingredients for self-love and self-sharing, we can reinforce these caring connections with the communication tools we'll pick up at Checkpoint 10, the next highway exit.

CHECKPOINT 10

Daring Difficult Conversations

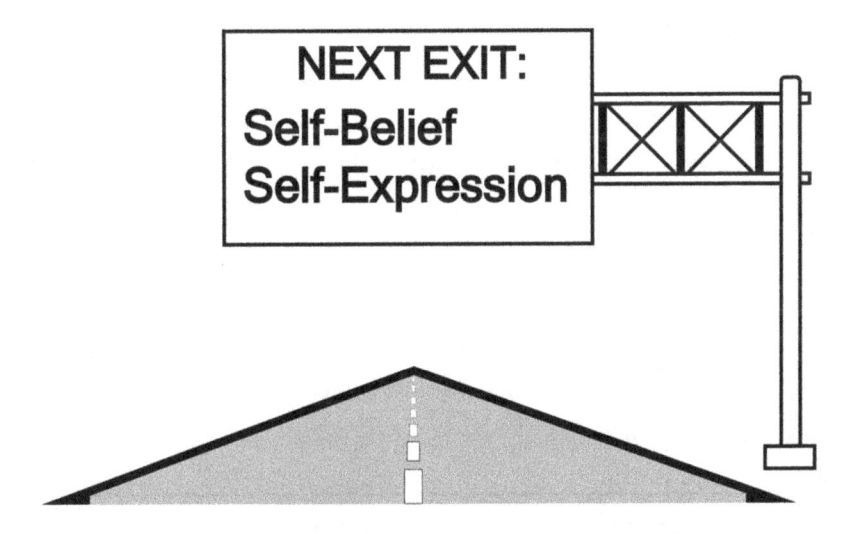

NEXT EXIT:
Self-Belief
Self-Expression

"Come to the edge," he said.
"We can't, we're afraid!" they responded.
"Come to the edge," he said.
"We can't, we will fall!" they responded.
"Come to the edge," he said.
And so they came.
And he pushed them.
And they flew.
— Guillaume Apollinaire

> *"The distance between you and everything*
> *you need is your language."*
> — Lisa Nichols

You have been plunged into deep inquiry and self-discovery on this road trip. You've done some very fancy driving — made some daring U-turns. The last few exits and construction zones have given you the chance to clear out even more limiting beliefs, paving the way for greater resiliency. I applaud you for facing your fears and trying out some new driving moves. Some of our deepest lessons occur when we show up vulnerably — when we show up clear in our "asks" — but without expectation or worry about the outcome.

At Checkpoint 10 in Part Three of this book, we'll revisit how the best moments for growth are those times when you take a leap of faith — believing you can soar. Those times when you lean into your pain and muster up the courage to have difficult conversations even though that's usually the last thing you want to do when you've been unfairly passed over for a promotion, you find out your teenager is addicted to oxycontin, or your partner has skipped off to Vegas with the contents of your joint bank account. All of these are true client stories.

If we connect to the lessons that we've learned along the way, our hearts remain open and curious even in the face of adversity. We believe in our ability to survive and are able to fully show-up and express ourselves. Openness to learning and tolerance for vulnerable conversations drives the powerful connections we discussed at Checkpoint 9 and fuels unwavering self-confidence.

Yes, building the confidence to express yourself in an emotionally intelligent manner is a critical skill for mental health resiliency.

Two of the best ways to build confidence are travelling and learning a foreign language. I observed these skills in ESL language edupreneur and well-travelled life navigation expert, Anesh Daya, after attending a webinar titled, How to Talk to Strangers. This webinar was also attended by international students from all over the globe who had moved to Canada and were not only trying to learn English and adapt to a new culture, but also trying to make friends and attend job interviews. How ironic that we spend our entire childhood being told not to talk to strangers, to be fearful of people you don't really know and to trust no one but yourself. Later, we're called upon to be fearless, take risks and network the heck out of everything.

I marvelled at the incredible resiliency these students demonstrated: adaptation, a willingness to be vulnerable, openness to difficult conversations, innate curiosity, optimism and belief in a brighter future. I can't think of a better way to learn this growth mindset than practising a new language — being completely exposed, vulnerable and certain to make mistakes. Talking to strangers means there's no room for fear if you want to express yourself and communicate your basic needs.

When I moved to Quebec in my twenties, I had no French language skills to speak of when I made the decision to relocate. I'd dropped French in high school, and since then I'd only ever used a French translator on business trips to Quebec. But, living and working in Quebec meant that I had to enroll in a French immersion language course and practise every day. So, I made an effort to get out of my comfort zone and risk being judged a fool.

I've never felt as unintelligent or exposed as when I attempted to use my newly acquired functional French in the real world. One of the funniest adventures in learning happened when a

Francophone friend, whom I trusted implicitly, helped me properly pronounce "poutine" — French fries with gravy and cheese curds — a Québécois Canadian staple. Unbeknownst to me, it was a set-up. Being armed with a little learning can be a dangerous thing. I waltzed up to the take-out counter and proceeded to order — in my most refined Québécois accent — two large prostitutes to go. I couldn't figure out why everyone was laughing and asking me if I preferred two men, two females, or one of each. I don't think my face has ever been such a bright shade of red. I said to myself, "That's it — I'm never speaking another word of French!"

Yet, resiliency is getting back up on that horse right after you fall and believing you will gallop again. So, instead of quitting, I held the unwavering self-belief that I could work for a francophone advertising agency one day. I kept practising and found myself years later presenting in French to the senior leadership team of a large multinational company. You see, anything is possible because "impossible" actually spells, "I'm possible!"

Confidence-Boosting Emotional Intelligence
Beyond language competency, what else makes you that resilient friend on speed dial? I'd hazard to guess you'd have a degree in perseverance and you're also very emotionally intelligent. This term was popularized in 2005 by Dr. Daniel Goleman in his book, *Emotional Intelligence: Why It Can Matter More Than IQ*, Goleman makes the case that we need to be keenly aware of how our emotions drive our behaviour in order to mitigate the positive or negative effect we have on others.[58] Good thing we picked up emotional self-regulation tools at our very first exit.

So, why does EQ (Emotional Quotient) matter more than IQ (Intelligence Quotient) and what's that have to do with our mental health resiliency? Well, I'm sure you're familiar with IQ tests primarily measured by our logical brain's ability to reason, memorize and retrieve data. Maybe you're still traumatized by those standardized IQ tests in school that often ostracized gifted students or misclassified others as having learning challenges. Whether the label was downright wrong or not, it often negatively affected a student's entire experience of learning and socialization. They were often bullied. Belief in their unique talents and abilities — outside academic measurements of success — was usually not modelled or even encouraged.

Now EQ and the newly recognized intelligence of CQ (Curiosity Quotient) or CI (Cultural Intelligence), namely, being openminded, willing to question your own beliefs and communicate with people from other cultures, are considered just as critical for success — if not more so.[59] EG and CQ are viewed as imperative to forming meaningful relationships, making sound decisions and being resilient in life. The great thing is you can grow and develop both your EQ and CQ over time. As lifelong learners on this road trip, that will help you get to self-fulfillment and self-enjoyment even faster.

Luckily, many of the mental health resiliency skills that you've been adding to your toolkit are also traits of EQ and CQ. Yes, I kind of planned it that way. So, you'll be pleased to know you already have EQ essentials like self-awareness, self-honesty, self-compassion, self-reflection, self-knowing, self-regulation, self-discipline, self-transitioning and self-soothing. Look at you go!

At this checkpoint, we'll add a couple more resiliency tools, using EQ and CQ to boost your overall confidence and ability to have those hard and heavy conversations. So, at this exit let's better equip ourselves with greater self-belief and self-confidence.

Then we'll practise self-expression by developing the crucial communication skills needed to build successful relationships before travelling to our final exit.

But first, what's self-belief?

Self-Belief + Self-Confidence = Resilience

Self-belief is the inner belief we feel deep down — the "I can do hard things" inner knowing versus self-confidence, which is the strength we project to the outside world. Both resiliency attributes promote our ability to bounce back from our life calamities. They also make us highly motivated to learn key CQ traits such as: hardworking, persevering and optimistic. When we're self-confident, we're better at creative problem-solving, too. We care more passionately about the "why" of what we do. That's an infectious attitude that inspires others.

Yet we all know that "look at me" boastful co-worker, who talks the "confident talk" doesn't really have authentic inner strength — genuine self-belief. Self-belief is an inner trusting that only comes from a willingness to take risks — a willingness to communicate your failures as well as your successes. As we've travelled along the mental health resiliency roadway we've also had to feel the fear and do it anyway, as Dr. Susan Jeffers recommends in her popular book by the same title.[60] That's a key pathway to test our immense human capacity and prove to ourselves that we will rise again. Experience is the best teacher.

The more dark packages that are handed to us, the more we acquire coping skills, which in turn builds our confidence resources arsenal to give us an empowered sense of control over our future life challenges. Then this cycle becomes a beautiful self-belief feedback loop. A continuous loop that helps us view and respond to future adversities in a novel way.

At Checkpoint 4, we practised looking at situations with a different set of eyes. Now, we can add self-belief to our reframing toolbox. For example, telling yourself, "I've been driving for years so I believe I'm a good driver," is a great start. But adding self-talk such as, "I'm confident I can safely handle any road conditions," and then actually proving it to yourself, is the best antidote. Real life risk-taking is often a critical component for reinforcing self-belief. The more you successfully drive on snowy roads or in crazy rush hour traffic, the more strongly you will believe that you're indeed, a very competent driver.

If we think back to the international students learning a new language, we can see how self-belief and self-confidence would grow exponentially once you're able to effectively navigate the world — take public transit, order food in a restaurant or get a bank account. Because little bursts of flourishing further motivate us to take even greater risks.

This willingness to fail speaks to the Japanese proverb *"nana korobi, ya oki,"* which means *"fall down seven times, get up eight."* Resilience is choosing to never give up hope, believing you will bounce back and striving for more. My friend Sensei Julie Creighton, (who has a 4th Degree Black Belt), describes resilience in the teaching of the traditional martial arts when she says, "On the surface all you see is fighting, but that is only the tip of the iceberg. When you dig deep there is self-healing; when you dig even deeper you find growth and when you go even further still there is strength to endure." Clearly, true resilience is earned, there are invaluable lessons in the pain, and the best teacher is experience.

GIFT BOX RESILIENCY TOOLS

Here are some strategies to reinforce your self-belief:

1. Set clear, specific goals for acquiring a new skill and chart out a plan to get there, with bite-sized steps and a way to track your progress (e.g., smartphone app).

2. Learn vicariously from role models. Observe and document what they do and how they seamlessly handle challenging situations. Try one of these strategies today and journal your observations.

3. Be open to seeking support and feedback — viewed as a sign of strength, not weakness.

4. Identify an aligned mentor to help you build an effective toolkit of coping strategies for difficult situations. This mentor could even be a co-worker, manager or success coach.

5. Keep seeking out people (e.g., friends, colleagues) who encourage risk-taking, get you out of your comfort zone and are doing the things you love to do. These people are your expanders. Write one person's name on a post-it note, stick it in a visible place and give them a call this week.

> 6. Be curious, keep risking and challenging your existing beliefs. Journal how you're growing, tackling hard things and succeeding. Celebrate your small successes.

SHOW UP FULLY — EMPATHIC COMMUNICATION

Now that we've looked at how to boost our confidence level, let's finally embrace the universal fear of speaking our truth, showing up as ourselves and having those difficult, authentic conversations. Yes, these are the kinds of discussions we usually avoid at all costs. I can see you looking for the next exit ramp. I understand why it might seem easier to just keep on driving your old "head in the sand" ostrich car. But, not speaking up for what we need, deserve and believe, means we cannot truly foster trust and intimacy in our relationships.

As a couples counsellor, I can emphatically say that limited self-expression is the main reason challenging relationships often go from "on the rocks" in the bedroom, to irreconcilably fractured in the courtroom. According to Dr. John Gottman, renowned University of Washington professor and couples communication expert, the problems underlying all conflict are essentially the same — we simply can't read each other's minds, so we need to learn how to adequately express ourselves.[61]

Yet here's the thing: the misunderstandings, stonewalling and communication challenges are not our fault. Most of us were never taught how to speak authentically and listen wholeheartedly in the first place. Yet, we can learn. It's never too late. Adding effective communication tools to your mental health resiliency toolbox will not only improve all your relationships; it will support your quest for living life with greater ease. And it's also the best route to find self-enjoyment at Checkpoint 11 — the final stop on our resiliency roadway.

To flourish and share your voice with others, you'll have to think beyond your own self-interest — "What's in it for me?" Instead, encourage all parties to contribute and succeed — "There's room for everyone" thinking. "Showing up" in this world means we allow other people to be heard, understood and validated.

Being equipped to have difficult, crucial conversations especially in the dark times can become your new resiliency superpower. Leaning into empathy fast tracks emotional intelligence and builds intimacy in all our relationships. It also means we have to withhold judgement and approach each situation with an open, win-win mindset. Easier said than done — especially when you enjoy finding fault with others as much as many of us do.

To show up fully, let's clarify the two types of empathy required:

a) **Cognitive empathy** is perspective-taking or being able to walk alongside someone and validate their emotional experience. For example, when someone is laid off, it's valid to worry about possibly becoming homeless.

b) **Affective empathy** is detecting the sensation or feeling we get in our body in response to another person's emotions and being able to mirror or state those feeling words back. For instance, "It sounds to me like you're feeling overwhelmed, angry and shocked." To do this you have to dig deep into your storehouse of memories to connect with a similar feeling you've had in the past. You might not get it right the first time but when you do, you will usually hear an emphatic yes with a deep sigh or sense of relief.

Let's face it, it's harder to have empathy for someone like a colleague who constantly complains. Being non-judgmental means you have to listen to your friend lament about a paper cut even if you've just been through major surgery, offering an empathic response for a seemingly insignificant wound. Instead of saying, "That's nothing, let me tell you from my experience something that's worth complaining about."

Empathy is knowing that all you need to do is give your undivided attention to a friend or colleague right here, right now, without thinking, "What's in it for me?", "Can I afford this time right now?" or, "Can't someone else help instead?" Giving your focused attention is especially needed if you've built up a "trust bank account" with a colleague and you're the one person they have chosen to confide in today.

Most importantly, to wholeheartedly show up you must practise active listening and be completely *present*. Being completely present means that you need to turn off your phone, stop all interruptions and make the person who is speaking feel like the most important person in the room. They deserve to have your focused attention. In this way, you're modelling how you'd like others to show up for you, too.

Active listening is the one small step you can start practising today to positively impact your own dark times and walk with others in their pain.

Stephen Covey's words ring true here:

"If I were to summarize in one sentence the single most important principle I have learned in the field of interpersonal relations, it would

be this: Seek first to understand, then to be understood. This principle is the key to effective interpersonal communication."[62]

So, it's called "active" listening because your only job is to listen and be completely focused on a speaker's words, tone, manner and body language. Believe me, when I get around people who raise my temperature, it is extremely difficult to not think about a rebuttal. Instead, I have to tell myself, "My only job right now is to hear what this person is saying and mirror back words and feelings until the person says "yes." They may not shout "YES," but you will witness an intense sense of relief when a person finally feels you really get what they have to say.

And honestly giving someone your full, undivided, presence is by far the best present you can ever give them. Better yet, if you've had a similar dark package yourself, tap into this learning and mirror back those same uncomfortable feelings and fears — that's affective empathy. In fact, imagine you have a magic mirror in your computer bag or purse. Your job is to pull it out and simply reflect back what you are seeing and hearing. That's how you go from the basement to the top floor of great communicators.

GIFT BOX RESILIENCY TOOLS

Knowing how to respond in an authentic conversation is very important because allowing someone to feel heard just might save a life. Again, this response models how you want others to listen to you.

Here are some responses to practise active listening and even support a friend or colleague in distress:

- "I'm here for you."
- "Am I getting this right?"
- "If I understand well, this situation makes you feel …"
- "Thank you for telling me that you're upset about …"
- "I'm not a trained counsellor so I'm not sure what to do or say to be helpful, but I want to get you to a trained professional who can help you cope with this."

Or you could simply say, "Let's work together to get you the help you deserve so you can get back to being the awesome person I know you to be!"

To be a good listener and express empathy, consider the following tools using this SOLER acronym:

- **S** — **Smile** and **Sit** down (focus only on the conversation)
- **O** — **Open** posture and **Open**-ended questions ("What do you mean? Help me understand why you feel that way.")
- **L** — **Listen** and **Lean** in
- **E** — **Eye** contact (eyes are the windows to the soul in most cultures)
- **R** — **Repeat** (paraphrase) and **Relax** (breathe)

EXPRESSING YOURSELF

Communication is a two-way street. Listening is crucial, but so is learning how to state your message effectively that is especially hard to do when you're feeling overwhelmed and in deep pain. That's where actions can speak louder than words. Did you know that when you try to express your attitude or feelings about a subject, the words you speak carry the least amount of significance?

According to American psychology professor, Dr. Albert Mehrabian, non-verbal communication (which is deeply rooted in the brain) is stronger than the literal content of a message.[63] It is also how humans determine whether a message is credible or not. For example, if you say, "I'm not angry," while stomping your feet and raising your voice, the message would not be perceived as credible or believable. So, the next time that you have to speak to someone about an emotionally charged or difficult subject remember the Mehrabian 7-38-55 Communication Theory:

- 7 percent of meaning is in the actual words spoken.
- 38 percent of meaning is paralinguistic (the way the words are said or tone/manner). Dale Carnegie's classic book, *How to Win Friends & Influence People* is a timeless reference for both verbal, non-verbal cues and effective communication tactics.[64]
- 55 percent of meaning is in facial expression and body language. I'd recommend renowned hostage negotiator, Chris Voss' book called, *Never Split the Difference: Negotiating As If Your Life Depended On It*, to better understand important non-verbal cues in all your communication exchanges.[65]

☕ COFFEE WITH CATHERINE

Let's sit down at the coffee shop and practise our self-expression skills by completing these exercises:

- **Try asking, "How are you today?" with or without voice inflection and body language** — Let's practise different ways to show your interest or disinterest by simply changing your tone of voice and body language (e.g., low grumpy voice or with crossed arms and little eye contact). Keep practising this technique with your friends and co-workers. For example, "How did you find your way out of this?" could have an inquisitive tone or an accusatory tone simply with your voice inflection.

- **Let's practise active listening using all your SOLER skills** — We can write out a script of a difficult subject you need to brooch with your friend, teenage daughter or partner. Remember to demonstrate you really care by paraphrasing, using empathy, body language and tone. Looking in the mirror when you practise your responses will really help you practise how to show genuine care and concern.

BE A HUMOROUS STORYTELLER

> *"Human life is basically a comedy. Even its tragedies often seem comic to the spectator and not infrequently, they actually have comic touches to the victim. Happiness probably consists largely in the capacity to detect and relish them."*
> — H. L. Mencken

One of the best ways that we can rock the critical skill of self-expression is by telling funny stories and laughing at our hardships. When dark packages are handed to us, dark humour is often one of the best survival and coping tools we have readily available. Through humour, we can see the silver lining in adversity a whole lot faster. Humour is like a cognitive-affective switch that has the power to instantaneously shift your emotional state. Now that's a superpower!

I vividly recall, after multiple surgeries and years of physio on my leg, a surgeon in emergency telling me that I might have flesh-eating disease at best, or osteomyelitis (deep bone infection) at worst. Both these conditions would require amputation of my lower leg. I thought to myself, "Are you friggin' kidding me? I didn't go through an entire pregnancy with a broken leg just to have it amputated years later!" Luckily, these proclamations were misdiagnoses. But, all I could think of after the initial shock of possibly losing a leg was, "Damn, this will make a really funny stand-up comedy skit one day!"

> *"First the doctor told me the good news: I was going to have a disease named after me."*
> — Steve Martin

Evidence shows that highly resilient people use storytelling and humour as a way to punch back at adversity. In my trauma work, alongside emergency service personnel, dark humour is the preferred tool to cope with agonizing events, relieve tension and vent feelings. Dark humour has also been found to enhance resilience during some of the most horrible events in human history. For example, during the Holocaust, victims reported using humour in ghettos and death camps to better cope with extreme trauma and adversity.[66] Perhaps that's because humour can completely distract us from our darkest moments and laughter relieves our pain. In my experience, it's also one of the greatest mobilizers for creative problem solving and hatching novel escape plans.

As we explored in Checkpoint 4, storytelling has always played an important role throughout history by informing us of the dangers in our world. Stories enable us to make sense of the world around us and find meaning in chaos. In all my work as an educator and speaker, I find the thing that people remember the most are not the pretty PowerPoint slides, but that one heartfelt, funny story.

I'm convinced storytelling is probably the best teaching medium of all. Storytelling is good for our bodies (by releasing feel-good chemicals) and good for our relationships (through forging strong, authentic connections with people). Above all else, stories that make us laugh — a good belly laugh — have been found to strengthen our immune system, boost mood, diminish pain and protect us from the damaging effects of stress. Storytelling that leads to infectious laughter supports good mental health, inspiring hope, releasing anger and encouraging forgiveness.

One of the best things that we can do is learn to laugh at ourselves and to see the absurdity and humour in embarrassing situations. When we laugh at ourselves, we can start to worry less about our adversities and stop obsessing about our flaws and scars. I'm not suggesting that when the pipe bursts and you're suddenly knee deep in water that you should laugh at your misfortune, but I bet there will be something funny about the situation after the fact.

I love collecting funny stories, and I have no shortage of them to keep my friends entertained.

"Catherine," my friend asked as the conversation at the dinner party started to wane. "Please tell us your search and rescue in Croatia story."

I often haul out the story of my lovesick fifty-something mother who was then dating a Croatian-born boyfriend with this house on the beautiful Adriatic coast of Croatia. The only minor issue was that she went to stay with him for a few months as the Yugoslavian war raged further south to Bosnia in 1992. The Canadian government strongly urged all Canadians not to cross the Serbia-Croatia-Bosnia borders. But, with my good friends, Randi and Michele (the latter, ironically, an army brat), we soldiered on because at that point it was a search and rescue mission for my dear Mom.

It's a fun superhero story about risk, danger, defying the government and parental disapproval. It's about a café getting blown up the day after you've been there, tanks, machine guns and grabbing the clothes on your back and a limited number of high heels — escaping across the Italian border to safety. Just being a rescue hero for your mom is a pretty cool story in itself!

In my real-life experience, these are the kinds of stories that are usually told by fun, awesome people who seem to have a knack for expressing themselves and rising above adversity. Hopefully, this strength will get me on the list for your next spirited dinner party! And since we know humour is an essential mental health resiliency tool with all sorts of excellent benefits, it's in our best interest to keep practising our storytelling skills. So, before we move on to

Part Four and make a final trek to Checkpoint 11, let's make sure we pick up some humour tools at the gift shop. Oh, and how about picking up some chocolate bars or red licorice? We've earned it!

🎁 GIFT BOX RESILIENCY TOOLS

If you don't find yourself laughing nearly enough, here are six ways to flex your humour muscle before heading to our final checkpoint:

1. Watch or listen to stand-up comedy while driving, walking or exercising. Watch funny shows and movies or read an amusing book.

2. Take a step back and be an observer in your own life by collecting funny stand-up comedy skits and material for a show.

3. Practise smiling. Even if you fake a smile (making the physical shape with your mouth), it can lead to increased happiness as your body releases feel-good endorphins.

4. Recruit "funny buddies." This idea is simple: if you have amusing people in your life, hanging around them is sure to make you feel better and release frustrations.

5. Practise laughter yoga that combines laughter and intentional yogic breathing (pranayama). It's a great way to release stress and put some giggles into your day.

6. Get playful! Unleash your inner child. Sing and dance with wild abandon. Jump in a puddle. Laugh with unrestrained joy.

7. Laugh at yourself. We all make mistakes, have quirks and goofy habits that are funny. Simply stop being so damn serious about everything!

"A person only plays when they are a person in the full sense of the word and they are fully a person only when they play."
— Friedrich Schiller

PART FOUR

GIVE

YOUR GIFTS IN DARK PACKAGES

"You have a choice. You can select joy over despair. You can select happiness over tears. You can select action over apathy. You can select growth over stagnation. You can select you. And you can select life. And it's time that people tell you you're not at the mercy of forces greater than yourself. You are, indeed, the greatest force for you."
— Dr. Leo Buscaglia

CHECKPOINT 11

Passion Meets Purpose — Living Your Dark Gifts

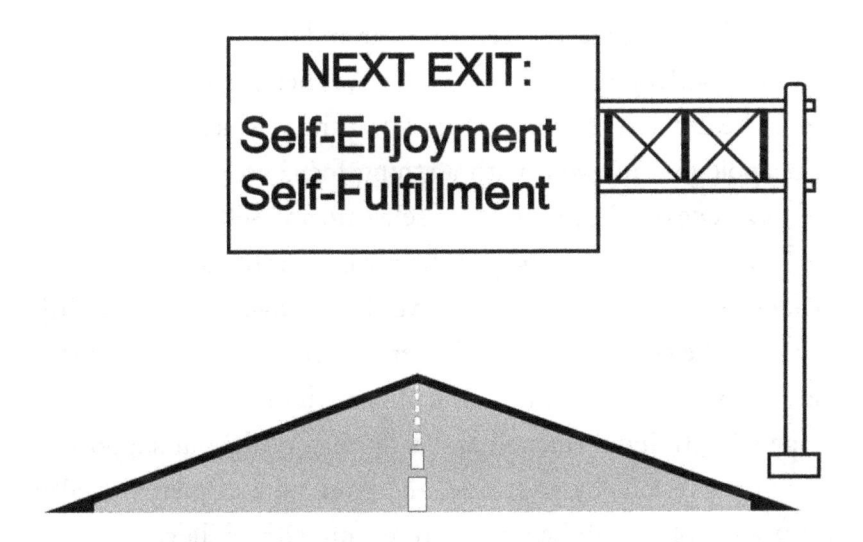

NEXT EXIT:
Self-Enjoyment
Self-Fulfillment

YOU HAVE PERMISSION TO LIVE MORE FULLY

"You can't go back and change the beginning, but you can start where you are and change the ending."
— C.S. Lewis

Congratulations! If you're still with me in this final section of the book that means you have already realized some significant post-traumatic growth. You've acknowledged, accepted and embraced some of your gifts in dark packages and illuminated your inner strength, newfound belief systems and appreciation for life. I'm sure just reading my real-life stories and those of my clients has been simultaneously traumatizing and illuminating. Let's face it — reality can be stranger than fiction.

If nothing else, I'm certain that from this day forward you will always put your car in park before reaching for the parking machine ticket — so many life lessons we've learned along the roadway.

Let's take a moment to marvel at how far you've travelled on this journey. To recap, we serviced your car and had it safety-checked to get you back on the highway of life. We then picked up essential mental health and resiliency tools along the way, learning how to be unapologetically you, with a strong focus on self-acceptance, self-forgiveness, self-compassion, self-care and self-love.

Now that you have the map firmly in your hands, you can get back on the resiliency road whenever life throws you a curveball. You have the skills to deal with overwhelming emotions like fear and loathing, your lifetime companions who love a good thriller peppered with inner turmoil and suffering. With your supportive pivot party friends by your side, and your suite of mental health resiliency tools, you'll be a force to reckon with. Believe me, your new spiritual transformation comrades will be seeking you out once you've returned from a few more self-partnered resiliency trips.

This final highway stop is about continuing to enjoy the ride and seeing yourself as a vehicle to make a difference in the lives of others. Ask yourself once again, "If your life were a book, how would you want your life story to unfold?" What are you so passionate about that you could do it for hours on end and never get bored? What comes so easily to you that it doesn't even feel like work? Or, as comedian Steve Martin so famously remarked in one of his comedy skits, "And I get paid for doing this?!"

I can see you giving me that "yeah, right" look. You're probably saying that famous line, "Some of us have to work for a living you know!" But here's the thing, if money can't buy you happiness, then what's the least amount of money you need to cover your expenses while living a life with purpose? I don't have the answer, but I'm working very hard on that equation myself.

In her ground-breaking book, *The How of Happiness*, positive psychologist Dr. Sonja Lyubomirsky wrote that only ten percent of happiness comes from extrinsic rewards like money, fame and status.[67] Of course, we already knew that. We've read how the happiest people in the world have found a way to combine their superpowers with their values and passion for a cause, person, or community — something outside of themselves.

Let's just agree that the journey of life is not about "getting" — somewhere, something, someone. Rather, self-fulfillment and self-enjoyment are the beautiful by-products of passionately following your bliss. A blissful, joyful state feeds your soul and often serves your highest good. As thirteenth-century poet Rumi so famously remarked, "What you seek is seeking you."

So, it's time to honour the bounty of your spirit — the gifts you're intended to give to the world. It's time to follow your North Star — the truth you've been unearthing all along. It's time to sit with me at the coffee shop and ponder:

- What has your heart been whispering to you when you're all alone in those quiet, meditative moments?

- What do you know deep within your bones, even in the smallest of moments and in the smallest of ways?
- What would help you create a purposeful, joyful life anchored in your own truth?
- What would feed your soul forever?
- What does the world need now and how can you have a powerful impact?

We're on a lifelong road trip here, so take your time. Just consider the goal of this last pit stop as pondering what will lead you to, "Yes, I found both joy in my life and brought joy to the life of others." These accomplishments were considered the determinants for a ticket to the afterlife in Ancient Egyptian teachings. The Talmud, an ancient Hebrew text, also lists three things you should do before you die:

1. Plant a tree
2. Nurture a child
3. Write a book

I just might be on track. How about you?
There are so many ways you can share your adversity lessons — your dark gifts — with the world. I invite you to ponder this "how" question as we edge closer to self-enjoyment and self-fulfillment on our road trip. Please take a deep breath and get very quiet. Make space now to listen for your wise inner voice as it speaks directly to you. There's power in simply observing and affirming that you are exactly where you are meant to be on this journey in this moment.

There is no sprint to the finish line. In fact, there is no finish line. That's just a mental construct we've created in our egoic minds to keep running, striving and exhausting ourselves. No more of that. We are not driving toward a destination but rather a state of being — a state of flow. Smile. Breathe in your wise inner spirit. Bask in your warm glowing light that was obscured by shadows for far too long. Feel your shoulders fall, your jaw relax, your forehead soften — that feels so much better, doesn't it?

All the things that no longer serve you on this roadway have already been tossed from the car window and the trunk is completely emptied. No more running, no more striving, no more scheming, no more fighting inner demons, no more comparing yourself to others, no more hustling, no more "I'm not good enoughs," no more caring what others think, no more catastrophizing and no more second-guessing. Phew! There's a clearing ahead, it's on the horizon. Can you see it?

As we round the corner toward self-fulfillment — the top of the resiliency roadway — I'd like you to set your GPS to whatever route is most meaningful for you. Your "why" — your life's purpose — the amazing way you can bring joy to others and serve the world. That's right. It's been inside of you all along — just begging to come out and play — to uncover your buried jewels. To quote author, Elizabeth Gilbert, *"Do you have the courage to bring forth this work? The courage to go on that hunt in the first place — that's what separates a mundane existence from a more enchanted one."* [68]

Simon Sinek, author of the book, *Find Your Why: A Practical Guide for Discovering Purpose for You and Your Team*, also believes that it's only when you understand your "why" that you will find the road you need to travel to get there.[69] Your "why" becomes your new reference point for all your actions, what you're curious about and what makes you feel passionate about your life. So, I challenge you to look at the work that you're doing right now — your relationships — and answer these questions:

1. Am I passionate about this job or career or am I just staying in this job out of fear because I need the paycheck?
2. Are you with a partner because you love this person, love yourself and feel adored and respected, or are you staying in a relationship because you're afraid of being alone or hurting them?

When you face and release resistance, your life starts to flow in the direction the universe has intended for you all along. And you've already picked up some tools to do just that. The Japanese use the term *ikigai* that can be translated to mean "a reason for being." This term means anything that gives a deep sense of purpose to a person's life and makes it worthwhile. It's what motivates you to get up every morning.

For a grandmother, her *ikigai* might be babysitting her granddaughter. For someone else, their *ikigai* might be simply supporting friends or volunteering at the local pet shelter. Maybe you've already realized true self-fulfillment as a parent, piano teacher, barista, loving partner or construction worker. That's wonderful because self-fulfillment often happens when we're bringing joy to the lives of others — your child, an acquaintance, a co-worker — with micro-acts of kindness and generosity.

What's important here is to stop squandering our time and energy in the endless pursuit of "the dream" that society has mapped out for us and to start pausing for long enough on this roadway to find a clearing — to ponder your own *ikigai*. Yes, it starts with just simply pondering — no more trying so hard to find "it." You don't need to keep busting through all the construction zones to arrive at some unattainable version of yourself. You can breathe a sigh of relief and be proud of yourself here and now.

Self-enjoyment is to be found in all of the quiet little twinkly moments — petting your dog, tickling a child, smelling the lilac blooms, holding your lover's hand or feeling a warm breeze. It's a very personal experience of living — the sheer pleasure of being alive that vibrates in you. Spiritual leader Michael Beckwith in an episode of Oprah's *Super Soul Sunday* podcast remarked, *"We're not in this world to get anything — we are in this world to let something unfold from within us."* I agree wholeheartedly. When you stumble upon your own "unfolding," there will be no disguising it.

I give thanks every day for my tumour — the dark gift I was given at thirty years of age. From that day forward, I realized that I could no longer work in an industry focused on frivolity and mind-numbing consumerism. I knew that I needed to do something more socially redeeming. I was motivated to make a positive effect on others, and on the world. I needed to be in a helping profession. I had to face my own mortality and ponder why on earth I had lived when my good friend — the mother of twin boys — had not.

Each and every one of us must determine what constitutes thriving and flourishing on the Mental Health Resiliency Roadmap. What does living a life with ease look like to you? What makes you smile from ear to ear? What makes you wake up every morning and say, "I am so blessed to have another day on this earth to do this one thing." It's often the simple and practical tools such as the RINGS daily morning routine that grounds you in gratitude.

It is my hope that you will continue to welcome the wisdom in your dark packages — the pain, the detours and the rejection — along the roadway. Freely and unapologetically choosing the exits that will make your soul sing. I encourage you to stop at as many exits and cafés as humanly possible. Maybe you'll decide to stop driving altogether, park your car and just take in the view for a while. Or maybe, like me, you'll pull over for long enough to write a book.

Whatever route you take, live your life like a bottomless cup of the very best coffee.

As we near the end of our road trip, I look forward to one last coffee chat and visit to the gift shop with you. Again, I want to congratulate you for the courage and resiliency you've shown on this tumultuous highway of life. Know that there are strategies and more downloadable resources at www.catherineclarkconnects.com to keep you learning, growing, rising and thriving.

Like you, I will be honing these mental health resiliency tools and working especially hard at self-care, self-surrender and self-partnering for the rest of my life. Painful experiences will always be part of my life and yours, but the mark of a purposeful life is how we accept, embrace and unwrap these dark packages and graciously gift them to the world. Taking responsibility allows us to evolve pain into empowerment, transmute suffering into strength and transform loss into opportunity.

If someone had asked me years ago, "What could you do for hours on end, never get bored and feel completely fulfilled?", I would have answered, "Talking to people, trying to figure out their motivations, helping them rise above adversity and writing good news stories." I've indeed found my North Star — my contribution that adds value to the world and holds great value for me. I believe whatever you're passionate about — your life legacy — is patiently waiting for you to emerge from the darkness and just be YOU.

I hope you will look back on this mental health resiliency road trip and realize that your darkest struggle was, indeed, the catalyst for your greatest transformation. Forgive yourself, make peace with the experience and release it. Best of all, celebrate your newfound, breakthrough self.

*Keep unwrapping your dark gifts and
watch your truest, most beautiful life unfold.*

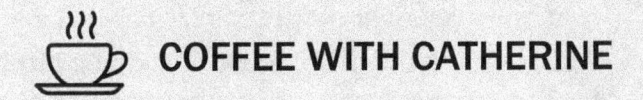

☕ COFFEE WITH CATHERINE

As we sit down for our last coffee pit stop, I have some important questions for you to ponder and capture in your journal:

1. How will you know when you're thriving and flourishing? Who would you be with? Where would you be living? What would you be doing?
2. Describe the photos on your vision board that paint a picture of what self-enjoyment and self-fulfillment mean to you. Scroll through the photos on your smartphone or on Pinterest for inspiration. What does a great day look like for you?
3. Let's say you're on an airplane winging its way across the Atlantic Ocean when the captain says the plane has engine trouble and is going to have to make an emergency landing. So, you grab your smartphone and send a message to a loved one to say goodbye and let them know about all the things you want to do with your life if you survive. What are the top three things on your list?

4. If you were diagnosed with a life-threatening illness, what trade-offs would you be willing to make to live? What would you happily give up or stop doing?
5. What simple blessing are you grateful for that you can enjoy right now (e.g., playing with my kids, visiting my aging parents, making a nice dinner, hiking a nature trail, and savouring a cup of tea)?
6. Taking all your best ingredients, write a recipe for a life well-lived. What are the stories that you want people to share about you? How do you want to be remembered? What's the legacy that you want to pass on? What's one action that you can take today to work towards that goal?

GIFT BOX RESILIENCY TOOLS

Please take a few minutes to revisit the many strategies that you have added to your mental health resiliency toolkit. Pick one strategy that you can start focusing on today. Write it down on a sticky note. Ask someone you trust for their help and support if needed.

- Do ONE new thing today that scares you. Fear + Excitement = Go Time.

- Say to yourself: "I'm thriving today not in spite of, but because of _____, my gift in a dark package." Write down or describe the dark gift that you're most grateful for today. How will you keep channelling the wisdom in this gift?

- Daily catch: Notice your feelings as they change throughout the day, while tapping into the thoughts below the surface. Adjust your perspective by substituting more, realistic thoughts and positive self-talk.

- Every day repeat to yourself: "I am good enough — I'm being the best version of me that I can be today."

- Give yourself permission to be uniquely you. Say out loud: "There is only one ME, and the world needs to hear my voice, receive my one-of-a-kind gifts and see ME shine."

HOW I OPENED MY GREATEST GIFT

As I stand on the shores of Lake Ontario
Feet planted firmly in the sand
Feeling relief from the inside out
I marvel at how far I've come
From Hotel Saskatchewan breakdown
Dark gift after dark gift
To penthouse Toronto skyline view
Sharing breakthrough stories

Healing painful wounds
On the rocky windswept shore
My deepest darkest bottom
Unwrapped with gritty hands
A loosening quicksand grip
Unearthing grateful me
Floating to the surface
Finding solace in the pen

Discovering dark soul flowers
Learning every word I write
Is paving a path for you
To brave your greatest fears
Trusting you enough
To reveal my darkest shadows
Knowing every step I take
Plants a garden for you to bloom

Now a published author
Celebrating this milestone
Basking in the sunbeams
Dancing in bright light
An abundance of roses
Still honouring the dark fall
On the greatest journey of all
Returning home to YOU

AFTERWORD – FINAL THOUGHTS

"The real voyage of discovery consists not in seeking new landscapes, but in having new eyes."
— Marcel Proust

It is my hope that this book has inspired you to look at the world with fresh eyes and to see that there's a gem hidden inside every hardship or painful experience. You have discovered the importance of a mindful morning routine, building in more self-care, reframing your self-talk, having empathic conversations and nurturing caring connections. If you feel better equipped to navigate the road ahead with more fearlessness, curiosity and compassion, then I have fulfilled my promise to you.

Yet inevitably, tomorrow may bring any number of life difficulties, catastrophes and suffering. None of us can escape adversity regardless of whether we're the CEO of a large company, a bus driver or a single mom with three kids — we must all take our turns. No self-help book can keep you from experiencing bumpy roads full of potholes, thick fog and stormy weather. Your Mental Health Resiliency Roadmap can help you find the on-ramps and exits needed to get through all kinds of road conditions, life-threatening accidents and close calls. Your resiliency toolkit will not only help you welcome misfortune but also aid you in feeling better and living better — *"grâce à l'adversité."* That's one of my favourite French expressions meaning "thanks to adversity."

The rest is up to you.

But here's the thing: it doesn't matter if I believe in you and the greatness you'll be unwrapping in your dark gifts. You must believe in yourself. It's your mindset that matters. It's up to you to keep honing your tools and adjusting your route because only you can decide to go forth and enjoy life. You can read more self-help books about resiliency, hire a life coach and post inspiring Instagram stories, but none of it matters if you don't believe in yourself.

The truth of the matter is that I didn't wholeheartedly believe in myself for most of my life. And it's ironic to think that I wrote a self-help book during a lockdown to help others heal from adversity, and in doing so, almost had another breakdown myself. Funny — not funny.

That's the interesting thing about life. Just when you think you're on the right track, you can find yourself flipped upside down in a ditch or a gutter. At least you get a fresh perspective on the world that you wouldn't otherwise have. And guess what? There are awesome tow truck drivers who can get you out of any ditch these days. The important thing is to figure out how you ended up in that dark gutter in the first place.

So, let's make this a "forever" road trip of continuous evolution — experiencing tough times, questioning, observing, surrendering, rising and unfolding as resilient human beings. Meaningful transformation is a life-long process: embracing the good, the bad and the darkest of packages. Breaking free of limited thinking to live the full spectrum of life — your authentic light — will definitely involve a few more resiliency road trips and stops along the way. That's to be expected.

Just know you can open this book and turn to a checkpoint whenever you need a reminder to step out of powerlessness and pain, and step into possibility and power.

Keep your hands on the wheel of self-discovery.

Keep unwrapping your dark gifts.

Drive with gusto to the pivot party.

And enjoy this wild ride called LIFE!

> *"A happy life consists not in the absence,*
> *but in the mastery of hardships."*
> — Helen Keller

> *"We are all in the gutter,*
> *but some of us are looking at the stars."*
> —Oscar Wilde

ACKNOWLEDGEMENTS

I am deeply grateful for all the incredible support that I have received in bringing this book to life. It was a difficult and emotional process to write a book for the first time, while in lockdown during a global pandemic. I promised both my children, "I would not die with the music still in me," and I always keep my promises. It's funny that the morning after I handed in the first draft, my daughter became worried that I had been hit by a car and killed, when I did not return home from an errand. She thought to herself, "OMG, Mom finished her book and then she died!" Now that would have made a tragically good story! I had actually risen early and visited my favourite French pastry shop to pick up two celebratory pains au chocolat. What was supposed to be a ten-minute trek became a forty-five-minute stop for a cappuccino, window shopping and chatting. Once I returned home in one piece, we had a good laugh about "curbing your catastrophizing!"

 I have a multitude of people and life experiences that have made this book a possibility from family and friends to people who have caused me pain and suffering over the years. Every one of you has played an important role in bringing this book to fruition. I thank each one of you. I send you all the compassion, light and love possible.

A heartfelt thank you to both my amazing children, Andrew and Nathalie. I'm eternally grateful that you chose me to be your mother. You are resilient, kind-hearted beings who really care about making a difference in the lives of others. You inspire me to grow and learn how to be the best version of myself every single day. Nathalie, thank you for your endless patience and artistic input on this book. Andrew, your discerning, philosophical inputs are appreciated more than you will ever know.

To my mom, Dorothy Clark, thank you for being my best friend, always believing in me and supporting me throughout all the dark gifts in my life. To my Rock of Gibraltar, course correcting sister, Wendy Marshall, I cannot express my gratitude for going "above and beyond" to always provide me with a safe place to land.

A giant thanks for the help and support of Laurie, my lifesaving best friend; Denise, my tried-and-true artistic confidant; and all my blessed soulmate friends who have pulled me out of the fire so many times they should have a firefighter certificate!

I am especially grateful to my amazing, talented circle of trusted advisor friends who not only cushioned my breakdown but also provided endless book writing encouragement, brainstorming everything from cover design to pictograms and providing fastidious editing support. I am blessed beyond measure to have these light beings in my life: Denise Cantlon, Anesh Daya, Warren Ellam, Tracy Shea-Porter, Laurie Stockton, Randi Tychsen and Karen Vanderheyden. A huge thank you is also reserved for my many brave friends and clients who have inspired me with their perseverance and strength throughout life's toughest challenges.

To everyone at Ultimate World Publishing, thank you for providing the supportive blueprint to breathe life into my dream of becoming a published author. I am grateful to my developmental editor, Maddie Johnson, whose insight and skills helped my words flow and kept me on track during those really tough writing days. Finally, thank you to my editors, Isabelle Russell, Tracy Shea-Porter, Alethea Spiridon, and Michele Wright, who skillfully helped me to the finish line. Last, but not least, thanks to my amazing proofreaders, Nancy Estey, Nyre MacPherson and Diane Rawlins.

NOTES

INTRODUCTION

Gilbert, E. (2016). *Big magic: Creative living beyond fear.* Riverhead Books, an imprint of Penguin Random House.

THE ROADMAP

Oliver, M. (2020). *Devotions: The selected poems of Mary Oliver.* Penguin Group USA.

Campbell, J. (2008). *The hero with a thousand faces.* New World Library.

CHECKPOINT 1: Acknowledge Your Gifts in Dark Packages

[1] Ekman, P. (2021, November 13). *Universal emotions.* Paul Ekman Group. https://www.paulekman.com/universal-emotions/

[2] Brown, B. (2022). *Atlas of the heart: Mapping meaningful connection and the language of human experience.* Penguin Random House Large Print.

[3] Maté, G. (2019). *When the body says no: The cost of hidden stress.* Scribe.

[4] van der Kolk, B. A. (2015). *The body keeps the score: Brain, mind, and body in the healing of trauma.* Penguin Random House.

[5] Brown, B. (2010). *The gifts of imperfection: Let go of who you think you're supposed to be and embrace who you are.* 160-1, Hazelden Publishing.

[6] CAMH. (2021). *The crisis is real.* https://www.camh.ca/en/driving-change/the-crisis-is-real

[7] CHEO. (n.d.). *Screening tools.* eMentalHealth.ca Resource Directory. https://www.ementalhealth.ca/index.php?m=surveyList

[8] Psycho Tests. (2021). *Beck's Depression Inventory.* https://psycho-tests.com/test/becks-depression-inventory

[9] Smetanin, P., Stiff, D., Briante, C., Adair, C.E., Ahmad, S. & Khan, M. (2011). *The life and economic impact of major mental illnesses in Canada: 2011 to 2041.* Risk Analytica on behalf of the Mental Health Commission of Canada.

[10] Tedeschi, R. G., & Calhoun, L. G. (1996). The posttraumatic growth inventory: Measuring the positive legacy of trauma. *Journal of Traumatic Stress, 9*(3), 455–471. https://doi.org/10.1002/jts.2490090305

[11] Stallard, P., et al. (2021). Post-traumatic growth during the Covid-19 pandemic in careers of children in Portugal and the UK: cross-sectional online survey. *British Journal of Psychiatry.* doi.org/10.1192/bjo.2021.1.

[12] MADD. (2021). *Statistics.* https://www.madd.org/statistics

CHECKPOINT 2: Accept Your Gifts in Dark Packages

[13] Germer, C. K. (2009). *The mindful path to self-compassion: Freeing yourself from destructive thoughts and emotions.* The Guilford Press.

[14] Seltzer, L. F. (2008). *The path to unconditional self-acceptance.* Psychology Today. https://www.psychologytoday.com/us/blog/evolution-the-self/200809/the-path-unconditional-self-acceptance

[15] Tolle, E. (2004). *The power of now: A guide to spiritual enlightenment.* Namaste Publishing.

[16] Doyle, G. (2020). *Untamed.* The Dial Press.

[17] Neff, K. (2021). *Fierce self-compassion: How women can harness kindness to speak up, claim their power, and thrive.* Penguin Life.

[18] Neff, K. (2011). *Self-compassion: The proven power of being kind to yourself.* William Morrow.

[19] Gilbert, P. (2010). *Compassion focused therapy: Distinctive features.* Routledge.

[20] Tirch, D. D. (2012). *The compassionate-mind guide to overcoming anxiety: Using compassion-focused therapy to calm worry, panic, and fear.* New Harbinger Publications.

[21] Kirschner, H. (2019). Soothing Your Heart and Feeling Connected: A New Experimental Paradigm to Study the Benefits of Self-Compassion. *Clinical Psychological Science*. www.psychologicalscience.org

[22] Luskin, F. (2010). *Forgive for good: A proven prescription for health and happiness*. HarperCollins e-books.

[23] Thomas, K. W. (2016). *Conscious uncoupling: 5 steps to living happily even after*. Yellow Kite.

CHECKPOINT 3: The Phoenix Fix

[24] Lerner, H. G. (2014). *The dance of anger: A woman's guide to changing the patterns of intimate relationships*. William Morrow & Co, an imprint of HarperCollins Publishers.

[25] Kushner, H. (2021). *When bad things happen to good people*. Bluebird.

[26] *Accelerated Resolution Therapy*. (2015, November 22). SAMHSA's National Registry of Evidence-based Programs and Practices. http://nrepp.samhsa.gov/ProgramProfile.aspx?id=7

[27] *How ART works*. (2016). The Rosenzweig Center for Rapid Recovery. http://acceleratedresolutiontherapy.com/how-art-works/

CHECKPOINT 4: Curb Your Catastrophizing

[28] Mahoney, E. (2009, September). *A Conversation with Dr. Wayne Dyer*. Natural Awakenings Magazine. https://www.drwaynedyer.com/press/conversation-wayne-dyer/.

[29] Rotter, J. B. (1954). *Social learning and clinical psychology*. Prentice-Hall.

[30] Burns, D. D. (2009). *Feeling good: The new mood therapy*. HarperCollins.

[31] Ellsworth, P. C., Smith, C. A. (1988). From appraisal to emotion: Differences among unpleasant feelings. *Motivation and Emotion. 12, 271–302*. https://doi.org/10.1007/BF00993115

[32] Fredrickson, B. L. (2013). Positive emotions broaden and build. *Advances in Experimental Social Psychology*, 1–53. https://doi.org/10.1016/b978-0-12-407236-7.00001-2

[33] Brown, B. (2015). *Daring greatly: How the courage to be vulnerable transforms the way we live, love, parent, and lead*. Avery, an imprint of Penguin Random House.

[34] Chopra, D. (2019). *Metahuman: Unleashing your infinite potential.* Harmony Books.

CHECKPOINT 5: Surrender It All

[35] Kabat-Zinn, J. (2013). *Full catastrophe living: Using the wisdom of your body and mind to face stress, pain, and illness.* Bantam Books.

[36] Ferriss, T. (2007). *The 4-hour work week: Escape the 9-5, live anywhere, and join the new rich.* Ebury Publishing.

[37] Shetty, J. (2020). *Think like a monk: Train your mind for peace and purpose every day.* Simon & Schuster.

[38] Wood, C. (2016). *The Labyrinth: Rewiring the nodes in the maze of your mind.* Austin Macauley Publishers.

[39] Hebb, D. O. (2012). *The organization of behavior: A neuropsychological theory.* Routledge.

[40] Tolle, E. (2004). *The power of now: A guide to spiritual enlightenment* (pp. 27). Namaste Publishing.

CHECKPOINT 6: Off-Balance

[41] Covey, S. R. (2020). *The 7 habits of highly effective people.* Simon & Schuster UK.

[42] Gazipura, A. (2017). *Not nice: Stop people pleasing, staying silent, & feeling guilty ... and start speaking up, saying no, asking boldly, and unapologetically being yourself.* Allen Publishing & Tonic Books.

[43] Doyle, G. (2020). *Untamed.* The Dial Press.

[44] Cole, T. (2021). *Boundary boss: The essential guide to talking true, being seen, and (finally) living free.* Sounds True.

CHECKPOINT 7: Challenging Change

[45] Bridges, W., & Bridges, S. (2017). *Managing transitions: Making the most of change.* Nicholas Brealey Publishing.

[46] Tedeschi, R. G., & Calhoun, L. G. (2004). A clinical approach to posttraumatic growth. *Positive Psychology in Practice*, 405–419. https://doi.org/10.1002/9780470939338.ch25

47 Duckworth, A. (2020). *Grit: The power of passion and perseverance*. Paula Wiseman Books.

48 Dweck, C. S. (2016). *Mindset: The New Psychology of Success*. Penguin Random House.

49 Seligman, M. E. P. (2018). *Learned optimism: How to change your mind and your life*. Nicholas Brealey Publishing.

50 Frankl, V. E. (2004). *Man's search for meaning: The classic tribute to hope from the Holocaust*. Penguin Random House.

CHECKPOINT 8: Living Through Loss

51 Kübler-Ross, E. (2002). *On death and dying; questions and answers on death and dying; on Life after death*. Quality Paperback Book Club.

52 Attig, T. (2011). *How we grieve: Relearning the world*. Oxford University Press.

CHECKPOINT 9: Deconstructing Disconnections – Cultivating Connections

53 Holt-Lunstad, J., Smith, T. B., Baker, M., Harris, T., & Stephenson, D. (2015). *Loneliness and Social Isolation as Risk Factors for Mortality: A Meta-Analytic Review*. 10:2: 227-237.

54 Hammond, C. (2015, May). *The Narcissistic Cycle of Abuse*. Psych Central Medically reviewed by Scientific Advisory Board.

55 Willcox, B. J., Suzuki, M., & Willcox, D. C. (2018). *The Okinawa Way*. Michael Joseph, an imprint of Penguin Books.

56 Oswald, D. L. (2016). *Maintaining long-lasting friendships*. M. Hoijat & A. Moyer (Eds.). The Psychology of Friendship. Oxford Scholarship Online. https://oxford.universitypressscholarship.com/view/10.1093/acprof:oso/9780190222024.001.0001/acprof-9780190222024-chapter-16

57 Riggle, N. (2017). *On being awesome: A unified 7theory of how not to suck*. Penguin Random House.

CHECKPOINT 10: Daring Difficult Conversations

58 Goleman, D. (1996). *Emotional intelligence: Why it can matter more than IQ*. Bloomsbury Publishing.

59 Friedman, T. L. (2006). *The world is flat: A brief history of the twenty-first century*. Farrar, Straus and Giroux.

60 Jeffers, S. J. (2007). *Feel the fear and do it anyway®: Dynamic techniques for turning fear, indecision and anger into power, action and love*. Jeffers Press.

61 Gottman, J. M., & Silver, N. (2007). *Why marriages succeed or fail: And how you can make yours last*. Bloomsbury Publishing.

62 Covey, S. R. (2020). *The 7 habits of highly effective people*. Simon & Schuster UK.

63 Casselberry, S. (1973). Silent messages. Albert Mehrabian. *American Anthropologist*, 75(6), 1926–1927.

64 Carnegie, D. (1936). *How to win friends and influence people*. Simon & Schuster.

65 Voss, C., & Raz, T. (2017). *Never split the difference: Negotiating as if your life depended on it*. Penguin Random House.

66 Ostrower, C. (2015). Humor as a defense mechanism during the Holocaust. *Interpretation: A Journal of Bible and Theology*, 69(2), 183–195.

CHECKPOINT 11: Passion Meets Purpose — Living Your Dark Gifts

67 Lyubomirsky, S. (2013). *The how of happiness: A practical guide to getting the life you want*. Piatkus Books.

68 Gilbert, E. (2016). *Big magic: Creative living beyond fear*. Penguin Random House USA.

69 Sinek, S. author, Docker, P. contributor, & Mead, D. contributor. (2017). *Find your why: A practical guide for discovering purpose for you and your team*. Portfolio Penguin, an imprint of Penguin Random House.

REFLECTIONS

REFLECTIONS

ABOUT THE AUTHOR

Catherine Clark has a Master of Education degree in Counselling Psychology from the University of Toronto, as well as certificates in cognitive behavioural counselling and crisis intervention. A highly respected mental health resiliency expert, Catherine has dedicated her life to supporting adults facing mental health challenges and life transitions. She is known for bringing her whole heart, humour and extensive experience to every counselling session, training workshop or senior leadership presentation, working tirelessly to break mental health stigma and promote psychologically safer workplaces.

Catherine is the Principal of Catherine Clark Connects, a boutique mental health consulting firm based in Toronto that specializes in helping individuals and organizations hold space for vulnerable conversations, build employee morale, foster engagement, encourage retention, and live more meaningful, fulfilled lives.

Catherine has extensive experience working on the front lines of trauma intervention including suicide prevention in the Canadian Arctic, crisis debriefing for major corporations and small group support for grieving mothers. She has facilitated hundreds of wellness workshops for multinational organizations on topics such as team emotional intelligence, work-life integration and embracing change. Catherine's keynotes reflect her talent for taking difficult topics and distilling them down with clarity, empathy and bite-sized solutions.

Catherine continues to support her clients with her Dark Gifts Mental Health Resiliency Platform and Pivot Party Program. Join an online Dark Gifts talking circle where you may be comforted, heard and understood — one human connection at a time. Book Catherine for a supportive Cat Chat coaching session, to speak on your show or to present a moving keynote to your audience today!

Visit www.catherineclarkconnects.com and explore:
1. Downloadable free tools: meditations, affirmations and Cat Chats (See QR code below)
2. Videos of inspirational speeches and keynotes
3. Workplace training and development offerings